P9-DXO-007

Ion Transport and Membranes

A Biophysical Outline

by A. B. Hope

Professor of Biology,
The Flinders University of South Australia,
Bedford Park, South Australia

BUTTERWORTHS LONDON
UNIVERSITY PARK PRESS BALTIMORE

THE BUTTERWORTH GROUP

ENGLAND
Butterworth & Co (Publishers) Ltd
London: 88 Kingsway, WC2B 6AB

AUSTRALIA
Butterworth & Co (Australia) Ltd
Sydney: 20 Loftus Street
Melbourne: 343 Little Collins Street
Brisbane: 240 Queen Street

CANADA
Butterworth & Co (Canada) Ltd
Toronto: 14 Curity Avenue, 374

NEW ZEALAND
Butterworth & Co (New Zealand) Ltd
Wellington: 49/51 Ballance Street
Auckland: 35 High Street

SOUTH AFRICA
Butterworth & Co (South Africa) (Pty.) Ltd
Durban: 33/35 Beach Grove

Published 1971 jointly by
BUTTERWORTH & CO (PUBLISHERS) LTD, LONDON
and
UNIVERSITY PARK PRESS, BALTIMORE

© Butterworth & Co (Publishers) Ltd, 1971

ISBN 0 408 70068 8
Library of Congress Catalog Card Number 76-148825

Filmset by Filmtype Services Limited, Scarborough, Yorkshire

Printed in England by Camelot Press, Southampton, Hants

Ion Transport
and Membranes

QH
601
H68

Preface

This book deals with some aspects of the relations between ions and living cells. Owing to the very great complexity of the simplest cell, the study of the way in which ions find their way into and out of cells is not at all advanced. Nevertheless the exploitation of the technique of following ion movements with radioactive isotopes, and the use of sophisticated electronic equipment, have led to a knowledge of some of the parameters involved; for example, the species and quantities of ions which move across excitable membranes, when the latter are suitably stimulated to give an action potential, have been measured in both animal and plant cells. In addition, at least one ion transport system has been tracked down to an identifiable enzyme.

The theory we have to connect ion fluxes with the driving forces is really very inadequate. This is due to the fact that membranes (which most, but not all, biologists think are responsible for regulating ion fluxes) are very thin structures, of thickness $\sim 100\text{Å}$, and made up of molecules to which only a general name can be given—for example, 'phospholipid'. In such a thin system even the use of the familiar integral calculus is suspect. There are certain formulas which are common in the literature of ionic relations, used with some or little justification to connect flux with ion activity and other parameters, or conductance with flux; these are developed and discussed in the early chapters. There is growing awareness among biophysicists of the relevance of the thermodynamics of irreversible processes. It is a truism that living cells are not at 'equilibrium' but happily often in a slowly changing 'steady state'. The approach via the thermodynamics of the steady state is a formalism but one that provokes thought about the interactions possible between ion fluxes. With non-living systems it has been possible to calculate frictional coefficients between ions, water molecules and membranes, which

151622

make some physical sense. With many living systems, on the other hand, the experimenter is faced with sets of Onsager coefficients that have no apparent relation with anything he can measure. Time and ingenuity may rectify this situation.

As befits an introductory text, the treatment is at a comparative and rather simple level. Where possible, however, quantitative comparison between theory and observation is attempted. Abundant references are given for further study.

Thanks are due to the following colleagues for permission to discuss unpublished results: G. P. Findlay, M. G. Pitman, H. D. W. Saddler, F. A. Smith, N. A. Walker and E. J. Williams.

List of Symbols

English letters

A	Area, cm^2
a	Chemical activity
c	Concentration, mol (or equiv.) l^{-1} (or cm^{-3})
$\bar{c}_s$	An average concentration of solute as defined in Chapter 2
D	Diffusion coefficient, $cm^2\ s^{-1}$
e	Electronic charge, $1 \cdot 602 \times 10^{-19}$ C
F	Faraday constant (96450 C equiv.$^{-1}$)
f_{ij}	Frictional coefficients
g	Conductance, mho cm^{-2}
j	A species of particles (often used as a subscript, e.g. z_j)
J	Electric current density, A cm^{-2}
k	Rate constant for an exponential process, s^{-1}, h^{-1}, etc.
$\mathbf{k}$	Boltzmann's constant, $1 \cdot 380 \times 10^{-23}$ J K^{-1}
L_{ij}	(Conductance) coefficients in Onsager linear equations
n_s	Mole fraction of a solute
P	Permeability, cm s^{-1}
$\mathbf{P}$	Hydrostatic pressure, atm, etc.
Q	Quantity of a chemical species in a phase
R	Gas constant, $8 \cdot 314$ J $mol^{-1}\ K^{-1}$
R_{ij}	(Resistance) coefficients in Onsager equations
$r_{(0)}$	Membrane resistance (at the resting potential), $\Omega\ cm^2$
S	Specific activity of a radioactively labelled solution, counts $min^{-1}\ mol^{-1}$, etc.
T	Absolute temperature
t	Time
$\mathbf{t}$	Transport number
u	Mobility, cm s^{-1} (V $cm^{-1})^{-1}$

V	Volume
$\overline{V}$	Partial molar volume, $cm^3\ mol^{-1}$
$\mathbf{V}$	Electromotive force
v	Velocity
v_{ij}	Relative velocity of particles i relative to j
x	Linear co-ordinate, usually normal to the plane of the membrane surface
X	Force, or electric field strength
Y	Radioactivity in a phase
z	Valency

Greek letters

α	A permeability ratio, P_{Na}/P_K, or mobility ratio, u_{Na}/u_K, or electro-osmotic volume flow, $cm^3\ C^{-1}$
β	Partition coefficient, or electro-osmotic permeability, $cm^3\ C^{-1}$
γ	Activity coefficient
δ	Membrane thickness, cm or Å
λ	Space or length constant, cm
μ	Chemical potential (μ_j of ion species j, etc.)
$\pi\,(\Delta\pi)$	Osmotic pressure (difference)
σ	Conductivity, mho cm^{-1} or (Chapter 3) a rate of flow of a substance relative to a membrane
τ	Time constant, s
ϕ	Net flux, $mol\ cm^{-2}\ s^{-1}$
$\overrightarrow{\phi},\ \overleftarrow{\phi}$	Unidirectional fluxes
$\phi_{oi},\ \phi_{io}$	Influx, efflux
Φ	Dissipation function, temperature. Entropy production $time^{-1}\ volume^{-1}$, or active net flux (Chapter 6)
ψ	Electric potential
ψ_m or $\Delta\psi$	Potential difference across a membrane, V or mV
Ω	Electro-osmotic flow coefficient, $mol\ cm^{-2}\ s^{-1}\ (V\ cm^{-1})^{-1}$

Contents

1. ION MIGRATION—SIMPLE THERMODYNAMIC
   TREATMENT   1

   1.1 Diffusion in open systems   1
   1.2 Separation by a membrane   2
   1.3 The forces moving ions   3
   1.4 The effect of specific membrane properties   5
   1.5 Unidirectional fluxes and the flux ratio   9
   1.6 Membrane conductance   11
   1.7 Permeation restricted to pores   13
   1.8 Compartments and isotope exchange   13

2. ION MIGRATION FROM THE VIEWPOINT OF
   STEADY STATE THERMODYNAMICS   21

   2.1 History   21
   2.2 Forces and flows   21
   2.3 Interactions   23
   2.4 Frictional coefficients   27
   2.5 Frictional coefficients and phenomenological re-
        sistance coefficients   31
   2.6 Effect of frictional interaction on flux ratios   32
   2.7 Appendix   33

3. EXPERIMENTS WITH NON-LIVING MEMBRANES   34

  3.1   Advantages of artificial membranes   34
  3.2   Ion exchange membranes   34
  3.3   Cellulose membranes   39
  3.4   Very thin membranes   40
  3.5   Applications to biological membranes   41

4. VISUALISATION OF THE STRUCTURE OF
  BIOLOGICAL MEMBRANES   44

5. MEMBRANE POTENTIALS AND RELATIVE ION
  PERMEABILITIES   49

  5.1   Introduction   49
  5.2   Permeability deduced from membrane potentials   49
  5.3   The physical basis of selectivity towards ions   56
  5.4   Conclusions   61

6. ACTIVE AND PASSIVE TRANSPORT   62

  6.1   The Nernst potential   62
  6.2   Nernst potentials for ions in *Nitella*   62
  6.3   Other cells   64
  6.4   Electrogenic effects   65
  6.5   The flux ratio criterion   67
  6.6   The short-circuiting technique   68
  6.7   Conclusions   70

7. THE ELECTRIC RESISTANCE AND CONDUC-
  TANCE OF CELL MEMBRANES   71

  7.1   History   71
  7.2   Relation between conductance and membrane pro-
      perties   72
  7.3   The relation between conductance and ion fluxes   74
  7.4   Conductance of 'internal' membranes   77
  7.5   Rectification   77
  7.6   Electrokinetic phenomena   81
  7.7   Conclusions   84

8. ION FLUXES   86

   8.1 Introduction   86
   8.2 Resting fluxes in giant axons   86
   8.3 Muscle fibres   88
   8.4 Plant cells   90
   8.5 The non-independence of potassium fluxes   92
   8.6 Conclusions   97

9. METABOLISM AND ACTIVE TRANSPORT   99

   9.1 Introduction   99
   9.2 The active transport of sodium   99
   9.3 Transport ATP-ases   102
   9.4 Light-dependent chloride transport in plant cells   105
   9.5 Potassium and sodium active transport in plants   106
   9.6 Conclusions   107

10. CONCLUSIONS   109

   10.1 Some unscientific generalisations   109
   10.2 Future research   110

References   112

Index   120

1

Ion migration—simple thermodynamic treatment

1.1 DIFFUSION IN OPEN SYSTEMS

At a plane separating two solutions of different concentrations, continuous collisions occur between the solute molecules owing to their kinetic energy of translation and rotation. These collisions result in a greater number of molecules crossing from the more concentrated to the less concentrated solution than in the opposite direction. A redistribution of particles takes place until the concentrations become equal, this process being called *diffusion*. At equilibrium, as with all such physical systems, the free energy of the whole is a minimum. Prior to the interdiffusion and levelling of the concentrations, work could have been obtained from the potential energy represented by the concentration difference; for example, a 'semi-permeable membrane' could have been interposed and fluid could have been raised in level. The free energy of a concentration difference is dissipated as increased entropy and waste heat during the process of diffusion.

Even at equilibrium, collisions do not cease: at the plane of former separation there are now equal numbers of particles crossing from left to right and from right to left. Such traffic could be demonstrated by 'labelling' the particles of one side with a radioactive or other identifiable isotope. The process of interdiffusion or self-diffusion would then be shown by the presence of some of the labels on the other side.

Description of these processes allows the introduction of some widely used terms. The traffic of particles across a plane chosen by the observer is the *flux*, given in units of amount per unit area and unit time. Hence, *net flux* is the net movement in a given direction.

The radioactive labelling experiment, provided that it is done correctly, allows an estimation of the *unidirectional fluxes*. At equlibrium, the net flux is zero (the difference between two equal unidirectional fluxes).

It is convenient to speak of the diffusion of particles in terms of the 'forces' that tend to cause it, and the resistance or opposition encountered by the particles during their motion. The force is related to a gradient of a function of the concentration called the chemical potential if the particle is uncharged, or to a gradient of the electrochemical potential if the particle is electrically charged. These terms are considered in detail below.

The resistance to the flux or flow is related to the 'friction' encountered during the movement of particles between those surrounding them in the solution. The reciprocal of this resistance is a conductance, in the general sense, and is related to the ease of diffusion, described by the *diffusion coefficient*. This is defined for the particular solute particles in a given solvent and, for moderate concentrations, is only slightly dependent on the concentration of the solution. A quantitative treatment of conventional diffusion can be found in textbooks such as that by Crank (1956).

1.2 SEPARATION BY A MEMBRANE

For the present a membrane will be defined as a thin phase of rigid material different from that on either side of it. In other words, the plane of separation described in Section 1.1 will be replaced by a material with properties different from those of the solutions it separates.

There are now at least two ways in which ions can pass through such a rigid membrane: by going out of solution on one side, into solution in the membrane and redissolving in the solution on the other side; or by passing via holes or pores (filled with water or solution) that are part of the membrane structure. The process as a whole is, in general, governed by the properties of *both the membrane and the outside solution*. There may be many situations, however, where passage through the membrane is rate-limiting.

The properties of the membrane which may influence permeation by ions are: its thickness; the solubility of ions in the membrane; the electric charge on the surface; the sign and density of this charge; the breadth, width and tortuosity of the pores; the electric charge in the pores; and the mobility of ions in the pores. A quantitative treatment of the way in which such properties govern the rate of movement of ions is still lacking. Certain properties, such as solubility and mobility, enter the theory in the way outlined below.

1.3 THE FORCES MOVING IONS

As with many forces in physics, the *gradient of a potential* has to be sought. For example, the rate of heat transfer is proportional to the gradient of temperature. The force on unit electric charge is given by the gradient of electric potential. The appropriate potential in ion migration is the *electrochemical potential*; the gradient of electrochemical potential is the correct force to consider.

It is worth looking at the factors in the definition of electrochemical potential, due to Guggenheim (1929). For an ion species j this is $\bar{\mu}_j$, given by

$$\bar{\mu}_j = \mu_j^0 + RT \ln \gamma_j c_j + z_j F \psi + P \bar{V}_j \qquad (1.1)$$

where μ_j^0 is the chemical potential in a standard state, R the gas constant, T the temperature in K, γ_j the activity coefficient, c_j the chemical concentration, z_j the valency (with sign), F the Faraday constant, ψ the electric potential, P hydrostatic pressure and $\bar{V}_j$ the partial molar volume. $\gamma_j c_j$ as a product forms the chemical activity a_j, and $RT \ln a_j$ together with μ_j^0 will be recognised as the chemical potential.

In this expression there are three and perhaps four quantities that vary as we proceed from a solution on one side into the membrane and out into the second solution. These are P, c_j, ψ and possibly γ_j. It is assumed that there is thermal equilibrium; T is therefore constant.

Discussion of the thermodynamic origin of the chemical and electrochemical potential is best left to specialists. There are at least two books that will help, one by Spanner and one by Katchalsky and Curran; both are listed in the References.

The force X_j on ions of the sort j can now be seen to be the negative of the gradient of $\bar{\mu}_j$, i.e.

$$X_j = -\operatorname{grad} \bar{\mu}_j$$
$$= -RT \, \partial(\ln a_j)/\partial x - z_j F \, \partial\psi/\partial x - \bar{V}_j \, \partial P/\partial x \qquad (1.2)$$

where x is the distance inside the membrane from one face of the membrane. The velocity of the ions subjected to this force is the mobility multiplied by the force, i.e. $u_j \cdot X_j$, and, finally, the flux ϕ_j in the x-direction is velocity times concentration:

$$\phi_j = (u_j X_j)c_j$$

$$= -u_j c_j \left(\frac{RT}{\gamma_j} \frac{\partial \gamma_j}{\partial x} + z_j F \frac{\partial \psi}{\partial x} + \overline{V}_j \frac{\partial \mathbf{P}}{\partial x} \right) - u_j RT \frac{\partial c_j}{\partial x} \quad (1.3)$$

This is a formidable equation, which can only be solved if $\mathbf{P}$, γ_j, c_j and ψ are *known* functions of x. That is, the way pressure, ion activity and electric potential vary as one metaphorically passes through the membrane must be known. What can be taken as known or measurable is the values of these variables on each side of the membrane.

It will be seen later that with a simplification it is possible to integrate Eq. (1.3). First it is essential to see what the conditions are for thermodynamic equilibrium. Considerations above suggested that at equilibrium the net flux is zero. Thus

$$\phi_j = 0 = -u_j c_j \left(RT \frac{\partial \ln a_j}{\partial x} + z_j F \frac{\partial \psi}{\partial x} + V_j \frac{\partial \mathbf{P}}{\partial x} \right)$$

Therefore

$$z_j F \frac{\partial \psi}{\partial x} = -\frac{RT}{a_j} \frac{\partial a_j}{\partial x} - \overline{V}_j \frac{\partial \mathbf{P}}{\partial x}$$

$$\int_o^\delta \mathrm{d}\psi = -\frac{RT}{z_j F} \int_o^\delta \frac{\mathrm{d}a_j}{a_j} - \frac{\overline{V}_j}{z_j F} \int_o^\delta \mathrm{d}\mathbf{P}$$

$$\psi^\delta - \psi^o = \Delta\psi = (RT/z_j F)\ln(a_j^o/a_j^\delta) - (\overline{V}_j/z_j F)(\mathbf{P}^\delta - \mathbf{P}^o) \quad (1.4)$$

The integration has been taken from the left-hand side (o) to the right-hand side (δ) of the membrane, of thickness δ. Even with a pressure difference across the membrane equal to 10 atm, the second term on the right-hand side of Eq. (1.4) amounts to less than 1 mV for most ions, because of the magnitude of $\overline{V}_j$. Thus, to a good approximation,

$$\Delta\psi = (RT/z_j F)\ln(a_j^o/a_j^\delta) \quad (1.5)$$

An equilibrium that results in a_j^o on one side and a_j^δ on the other side of the membrane *also* results in a potential difference $\Delta\psi$. Conversely, if a p.d. $\Delta\psi$ is established, the particular ion activity ratio given by Eq. (1.5) must follow. Equation (1.5) is Nernst's equation for the equilibrium potential difference for ions j.

The Nernst equation is the basis of attempts to separate the observed fluxes in living systems into those that follow from the observed 'physical' or 'passive' forces as described above, and those fluxes that are not expected on these grounds. The unexpected fluxes are probably dependent on metabolic activity in the cell—they are 'active' fluxes. A description of this application of the Nernst equation is given in Chapter 6.

1.4 THE EFFECT OF SPECIFIC MEMBRANE PROPERTIES

1.4.1 A specific electric field within the membrane

For the purpose of integrating Eq. (1.3), Goldman (1943) made the arbitrary assumption that the electric field within the membrane is a constant. This is equivalent to postulating a linear potential gradient. Thus,

$$\partial\psi/\partial x = (\psi^\delta - \psi^\circ)/\delta = \Delta\psi/\delta \tag{1.6}$$

The equation for the net flux of an ion when the membrane has a constant field is usually obtained in the following way. Starting with Eqs. (1.3) and (1.6), neglect the pressure gradient and put $\partial\gamma/\partial x = 0$. Then,

$$\phi_j = -u_j RT\, \partial c_j/\partial x - u_j c_j z_j F \Delta\psi/\delta$$

therefore

$$\int_o^\delta dx = -u_j RT \int_o^\delta dc_j/(\phi_j + u_j c_j z_j F\Delta\psi/\delta)$$

$$= \frac{\delta RT}{z_j F\Delta\psi} \ln \frac{\phi_j + u_j c_j^\circ z_j F\Delta\psi/\delta}{\phi_j + u_j c_j^\delta z_j F\Delta\psi/\delta}$$

Rearranging,

$$\phi_j = -\frac{u_j z_j F\Delta\psi}{\delta} \frac{c_j^\circ - c_j^\delta \exp(z_j F\Delta\psi/RT)}{1 - \exp(z_j F\Delta\psi/RT)} \tag{1.7}$$

where c_j° and c_j^δ are concentrations just within the membrane. If there is reason to believe that these differ from the concentrations of the bathing solutions on sides o and δ, it is usual to put $c_j^\circ = \beta_j c_j^{\circ-}$, $c_j^\delta = \beta_j c_j^{\delta+}$, where $c_j^{\circ-}$ and $c_j^{\delta+}$ are the concentrations outside the membrane and β_j is a partition coefficient or expression of relative solubility of the ions j in the membrane. Alternatively, it might be appropriate to reintroduce activities by putting $c_j^\circ = \beta_j a_j^{\circ-}$, etc. One of the discouraging things about trying to apply Eq. (1.7) to biological membranes is that some of the quantities are unknown. In particular, mobilities and solubilities are uncertain, and δ is usually taken as the thickness of certain dark lines in electron micrographs of very dead cells. When these uncertainties intrude, the parameters u_j and δ

are lumped together to form P_j, a permeability coefficient, with units cm s^{-1}:

$$\phi_j = -\frac{P_j z_j F \Delta\psi}{RT} \frac{c_j^o - c_j^\delta \exp(z_j F \Delta\psi/RT)}{1 - \exp(z_j F \Delta\psi/RT)} \qquad (1.8)$$

where $P_j = u_j RT/\delta$.

The graphs in Fig. 1.1 illustrate how the net flux of a monovalent cation would be expected to vary with varying (electric) potential difference (p.d.) with several different concentrations, all other

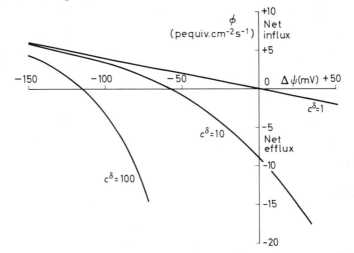

Fig. 1.1   *The net flux (ϕ) of a univalent cation through a membrane across which there is a potential difference $\Delta\psi$, according to the Goldman equation (Eq. 1.8). P_j has been taken as 10^{-6} cm s^{-1}, c^o constant at 1 mequiv. l^{-1} and c^δ given the three values indicated: 1, 10 and 100 mequiv. l^{-1}. ψ_j, the equilibrium potential, is the potential where the net flux is zero and occurs at 0, -58 and -116 mV, respectively*

conditions being assumed constant. Naturally Eq. (1.8) reduces to Nernst's equation when $\phi_j = 0$.

If the membrane is permeable to more than one ion, under conditions of zero electric current between sides o and δ it is possible to express the p.d. in terms of the concentrations and permeabilities. Thus, for the three ion species K$^+$, Na$^+$ and Cl$^-$,

$$\psi_m = 58 \log_{10} \frac{P_K K^o + P_{Na} Na^o + P_{Cl} Cl^\delta}{P_K K^\delta + P_{Na} Na^\delta + P_{Cl} Cl^o}$$

$$= 58 \log_{10} \frac{K^o + (P_{Na}/P_K) Na^o + (P_{Cl}/P_K) Cl^\delta}{K^\delta + (P_{Na}/P_K) Na^\delta + (P_{Cl}/P_K) Cl^o} \qquad (1.9)$$

where $\psi_m = \Delta\psi$ of previous equations and K^o, Na^o, Cl^o, K^δ, Na^δ and Cl^δ are appropriate concentrations. These are the Goldman or Hodgkin–Katz equations, widely used in interpreting membrane potential differences.

1.4.2 Conditions for a constant ratio of permeability coefficients

A constant ratio of the permeabilities in Eq. (1.9) follows from their definition through the Goldman flux equation. The coefficients here are themselves constant.

Without the assumption of a constant field there are some special circumstances in which the ratios P_{Na}/P_K, P_{Cl}/P_K, etc., are constant. Sandblom and Eisenman (1967) showed that when the ionic strengths of solutions on both sides of a membrane are similar, an equation like (1.9) with constant permeability ratios is appropriate.

When the membrane is permeable to ions of one sign only, a reduced form of Eq. (1.9) is correct for the p.d. No assumption is needed about the membrane field in this instance, either. This was also demonstrated by Sandblom and Eisenman (1967) but can be derived along these lines.

When the membrane is permeable to potassium and sodium ions only $(z_j = +1)$,

$$\phi_K = -c_K u_K \left(\frac{RT}{c_K} \frac{\partial c_K}{\partial x} + F \frac{\partial \psi}{\partial x} \right)$$

$$\phi_{Na} = -c_{Na} u_{Na} \left(\frac{RT}{c_{Na}} \frac{\partial c_{Na}}{\partial x} + F \frac{\partial \psi}{\partial x} \right)$$

In the absence of external current, $\phi_K + \phi_{Na} = 0$;

therefore

$$\frac{\partial}{\partial x} (u_K c_K + u_{Na} c_{Na}) + \frac{F}{RT} (u_K c_K + u_{Na} c_{Na}) \frac{\partial \psi}{\partial x} = 0$$

therefore $\qquad \left[\ln(u_K c_K + u_{Na} c_{Na}) \right]_o^\delta = \left[-\frac{F}{RT} \psi \right]_o^\delta$

therefore $\qquad \psi^\delta - \psi^o = \psi_m = \frac{RT}{F} \ln \frac{u_K c_K^o + u_{Na} c_{Na}^o}{u_K c_K^\delta + u_{Na} c_{Na}^\delta}$ $\qquad$ (1.10)

As before, a partition coefficient could be inserted by setting $c_j^o = \beta_j a_j^{o-}$, etc. β_j would be absorbed into a new permeability coefficient different from that in the Goldman equation. The ratio of the coefficients P_{Na}/P_K is the same in both treatments; thus, a useful form of (1.10) is

$$\psi_m = \frac{RT}{F} \ln \frac{a_K^{o-} + \alpha a_{Na}^{o-}}{a_K^{\delta+} + \alpha a_{Na}^{\delta+}} \tag{1.11}$$

where $\alpha = u_{Na}/u_K = P_{Na}/P_K$ is a constant.

1.4.3 A fixed charge within the membrane

If attention is first directed to the two interfaces between the solutions and the membrane, it is apparent that there will be interfacial components of the total p.d. due to the charges on the membrane surfaces. The surfaces can be assumed to come quickly to equilibrium

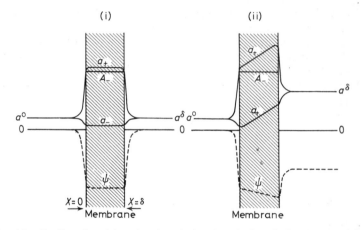

Fig. 1.2   *Profiles of activity of cations* (a_+), *anions* (a_-) *and electric potential* (ψ) *near a membrane containing negative charges* A_-. *In* (i) *the activities on each side are equal and in* (ii) $a^\delta > a^o$

with the respective adjoining solutions, leaving a diffusion process going on steadily *within* the membrane. For example, any of the profiles of potential drawn in Fig. 1.2 might be found.

   If the membrane is so highly charged that co-ions are effectively excluded, a linear potential gradient occurs again *within* the membrane (Karreman and Eisenman, 1962), but not of course from one solution to the other via the membrane. A simple theory for the p.d. and ionic distribution between solutions and charged surfaces and phases is given elsewhere (Briggs, Hope and Robertson, 1961).

A key relationship between local ionic activity and local potential at any plane x between $x = -\infty$ and $x = 0$ or between $x = \delta$ and $x = +\infty$ is the Boltzmann equation:

$$a_j^x = a_j^b \exp(-z_j F \psi^x / RT) \tag{1.12}$$

where a_j^b is the activity in the bulk solution (at $x = -\infty$ on the left-hand side or at $x = +\infty$ on the right-hand side). ψ^x is then referred to the appropriate bulk phase.

Equation (1.12) means that approaching a negatively charged surface the local cation activity is found to be greater than the activity some distance away, and increases by a factor of ten for every 58 mV by which the potential is lowered. Conversely, the anion activity is lowered at the same rate. The effect of a charged surface is thus analogous to that of a charged phase in causing an increase of counterion, and diminution of co-ion activity, compared with the solution outside. Equation (1.12) could have been derived by assuming equality of electrochemical potential between the bulk phases and planes $\delta < x < \infty$, $-\infty < x < 0$ up to the surface. At the surfaces themselves it will be assumed for the present that the 'solubility constant' relating activity just outside the membrane to that just within it is unity. Then we can write for the surface activities

$$a_j^{o+} = a_j^{o-} = a^o = a_j^{-\infty} \exp(-z_j F \psi^o / RT) \tag{1.13a}$$

$$a_j^{\delta+} = a_j^{\delta-} = a^\delta = a_j^{+\infty} \exp(-z_j F \psi^\delta / RT) \tag{1.13b}$$

ψ^o is now the potential referred to $\psi^{-\infty} = 0$ and ψ^δ is referred to $\psi^{+\infty} = 0$. Within the membrane there will be a diffusion potential depending on the ionic mobilities within it and on the activities.

1.5 UNIDIRECTIONAL FLUXES AND THE FLUX RATIO

Referring again to Eq. (1.3), the general equation for the net flux of an ion species moving passively, by neglecting $\partial \gamma_j / \partial x$ and $\partial P / \partial x$ we have

$$\phi_j = -u_j RT \frac{\partial c_j}{\partial x} - u_j c_j z_j F \frac{\partial \psi}{\partial x}$$

with the boundary conditions $c_j = c_j^0$, c_j^δ at $x = o$, δ and $\psi = o$, ψ_m at $x = o$, δ, respectively.

If we use as an integrating factor $\exp(z_jF\psi/RT)$:

$$\phi_j \int_0^\delta \exp(z_jF\psi/RT)\,dx$$

$$= -u_jRT \int_0^\delta \left[\frac{z_jF}{RT} \exp(z_jF\psi/RT) \right.$$

$$\left. + \frac{dc_j}{d\psi} \exp(z_jF\psi/RT) \right] d\psi$$

$$= -u_jRT[c_j \exp(z_jF\psi/RT)]_0^\delta$$

$$= u_jRT\,[c_j^0 - c_j^\delta \exp(z_jF\psi_m/RT)]$$

therefore

$$\phi_j = \frac{u_jRT\,[c_j^0 - c_j^\delta \exp(z_jF\psi_m/RT)]}{\int_0^\delta \exp(z_jF\psi/RT)\,dx} \tag{1.14}$$

Now c_j^0, c_j^δ, ψ_m strictly refer to quantities just within the membrane. What we know or measure is the corresponding quantities in the solutions on each side. Provided that the surfaces come to equilibrium with the solutions quickly, compared to the rate of diffusion within the membrane, it is permissible to put the solution quantities in Eq. (1.14), i.e.

$$\phi_j = \frac{\beta u_jRT\,[a_j^{0-} - a_j^{\delta+} \exp(z_jF\psi_m/RT)]}{\int_0^\delta \exp(z_jF\psi/RT)\,dx} \tag{1.15}$$

where now $\psi_m = \psi^{\delta+} - \psi^{0-}$.

Since the way ψ may vary with x is not known or assumed here, it is not possible to complete the integration. However, a most useful expression for the ratio of the unidirectional fluxes can be obtained as follows. The net flux is the difference between the influx and efflux: $\phi_j = \overrightarrow{\phi_j} - \overleftarrow{\phi_j}$. It is conventional to identify the unidirectional fluxes with the two terms in Eq. (1.15), because, in a sense, when influx is measured, the outside solution is labelled and the radioactivity of the inside is, initially at any rate, zero. The converse is true for a measurement of efflux. Hence,

$$\overrightarrow{\phi_j} = \frac{\beta u_jRT\,a_j^{0-}}{\int_0^\delta \exp(z_jF\psi/RT)\,dx}$$

and

$$\overleftarrow{\phi_j} = \frac{\beta u_jRT\,a_j^{\delta+} \exp(z_jF\psi_m/RT)}{\int_0^\delta \exp(z_jF\psi/RT)\,dx}$$

thus

$$\overrightarrow{\phi_j}/\overleftarrow{\phi_j} = (a_j^{0-}/a_j^{\delta+})\exp(-z_jF\psi_m/RT) \tag{1.16}$$

This expression was derived by both Ussing (1949) and Teorell (1949). At equilibrium $\psi_m = \psi_j$ (the Nernst potential) and the flux is unity (because $\psi_j = (RT/z_jF)\ln a_j^{o-}/a_j^{\delta+}$), but for other potential differences the ratio is not unity.

Equation (1.16) provides a useful test for passive, independent migration of ions (but see Chapters 2 and 3). The experimentally found flux ratio is compared with that expected from the observed ratio of activities, and ψ_m.

1.6 MEMBRANE CONDUCTANCE

1.6.1 Definitions of conductance

Several definitions of conductance are in use, all expressing the rate of change of net current flowing through the membrane in response to a change in potential difference across it. Thus,

$$g_m = \partial J/\partial \psi_m \text{ is the slope conductance} \qquad (1.17)$$

$$g'_m = \Delta J/\Delta \psi_m \text{ is the chord conductance} \qquad (1.18)$$

When the p.d. is changed from the resting level, at which the net fluxes of all the ions not at equilibrium add up to zero, the net fluxes of each of the ions changes, the membrane conductance can be regarded as a sum of the partial conductances, $g_j = F(\partial\phi_j/\partial\psi_m)$, corresponding to (1.17) or $g'_j = \Delta J_j/(\psi_m - \psi_j)$ (Hodgkin and Huxley, 1952), with

$$g_m = \sum_j g_j$$

Theoretical expressions for the conductance start with relations between net flux and potential. It has been noted already that it is impossible to integrate the general flux equation (1.3) without simplifying assumptions. The Goldman equation (1.8) is the usual relation assumed between net flux and potential. Planck's assumption of microscopic electroneutrality at all places within the membrane is a further plausible way of proceeding (Hope and Walker, 1961; Rosenberg, 1969) but leads to more complex equations for both p.d. and resistance.

1.6.2 The resting conductance when the Goldman assumption is used

If we restrict consideration to monovalent ions only, the membrane resting conductance comes from differentiation of the net flux for each contributing ion, addition of the partial conductances and use of the relation

$$\psi_m = \frac{RT}{F} \ln \frac{C_+^o + C_-^\delta}{C_+^\delta + C_-^o},$$

another form of Eq. (1.9, where $C = \sum_j P_j a_j$ for the cations and anions separately, in each phase. By use of Eq. (1.8) for ϕ_j, with the appropriate conventions about the sign of the currents, it may be shown that

$$g_0 = \frac{F^2 \ln \dfrac{C_+^o + C_-^\delta}{C_+^\delta + C_-^o}}{RT \left[\dfrac{1}{C_+^o + C_-^\delta} - \dfrac{1}{C_+^\delta + C_-^o} \right]} \tag{1.19}$$

1.6.3 The chord conductance

A general equation for the chord conductance is more complicated than (1.19) above. A feasible way of calculating this conductance would be to compute ϕ_j for a range of p.d.s, the parameters P_j, $a_j^{o\,\delta}$ being used, for each of ions of interest. Hence, on addition to get the total net flux or current at various ψ_m, g'_m follows from Eq. (1.18).

If the membrane is permeable to monovalent cations only, then it may be shown that

$$g'_m = \frac{F^2 \psi_m C_+^o \left[1 - \exp (F \Delta\psi_m/RT) \right]}{RT \Delta\psi_m [1 - \exp F\psi_m/RT]} \tag{1.20}$$

1.6.4 Conductance and flux at the Nernst potential

There is a simple equation for the partial conductance expected from an observed unidirectional flux, when the Nernst condition for electrochemical equilibrium is satisfied for that ion species, and when influx and efflux are independent of each other and of other fluxes (Hodgkin, 1951).

Since $J_j = z_j F(\overrightarrow{\phi}_j - \overleftarrow{\phi}_j)$,

$$g_j = \partial J_j/\partial \psi_m = z_j F \frac{\partial}{\partial \psi_m}\left[\overleftarrow{\phi}_j\left(\frac{\overrightarrow{\phi}_j}{\overleftarrow{\phi}_j} - 1\right)\right]$$

whence, from Eq. (1.16), $g_j = (z_j^2 F^2/RT)\phi_j$, since $\overrightarrow{\phi}_j = \overleftarrow{\phi}_j = \phi_j$ when $\psi_m = \psi_j$. For example, a flux of 1 pmol cm^{-2} s^{-1} of a mono-valent ion contributes 3·8 μmho cm^{-2} partial conductance, at 20°C. If this were the only flux, the membrane resistance would be 260 kΩcm^2.

1.7 PERMEATION RESTRICTED TO PORES

This restriction introduces the likelihood of strong interaction between ions and ions, and ions and water. That between ions and the membrane material has already been expressed in P_j or u_j above. Interactions are best dealt with through the thermodynamics of the steady state (of irreversible processes) and so are left until the next chapter. In this chapter simple models of ions moving *independently* have been considered, such as might be the case if ions dissolved in the membrane material to form a dilute solution.

1.8 COMPARTMENTS AND ISOTOPE EXCHANGE

We now consider the way in which model systems are expected to behave in relation to the uptake or elution of radioactive label. It will be necessary to refer to the equations and graphs during the discussion of the fluxes of ions in cells, in Chapter 8.

1.8.1 One compartment

Consider first an inner closed space, of volume V and surface area A, having a concentration c_i of substance j inside. This compartment has a thin boundary (membrane), which is assumed to control the rate of passage of the substance considered into and out of the space. This might be a reasonable first model for some animal cells. Diffusion outside and inside the compartment is rapid, so that the gradient of j or of a radioactive version called j* is entirely across the surface boundary of the compartment.

If there are constant unidirectional fluxes of j across this boundary $\phi_{oi} = \phi_{io} = \phi$, we wish to know how the radioactivity of the compartment builds up following the introduction of isotope outside, and how it subsequently decreases on the reduction of the specific activity outside to zero. Then, these rates being known, it is possible to calculate the flux from a tracer experiment.

From the terms defined in Fig. 1.3:

(a) For uptake, $S_i = Y_i = 0$ at $t = 0$; $S_o = $ const.

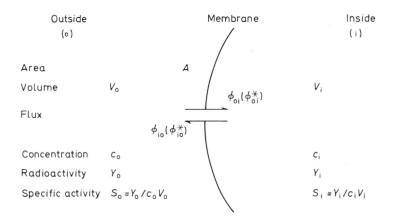

Fig. 1.3 *The quantities considered in relating radioactivity or specific activity to time, during the course of labelling or eluting a single compartment 'i'. Fluxes usually in* mol cm^{-2} s^{-1}, *concentrations in* mol cm^{-3}, *radioactivity in* counts min^{-1}, *and specific activity in* counts min^{-1} mol^{-1}.

Then
$$\frac{dY_i}{dt} = A(\phi_{oi}^* - \phi_{io}^*)$$

$$= A(S_o\phi_{oi} - S_i\phi_{io}) = (S_o - S_i)\phi \cdot A$$

or
$$\frac{dS_i}{dt} = \phi A(S_o - S_i)/c_iV_i$$

whence, by use of the initial conditions defined,

$$S_i = S_o[1 - \exp(-\phi At/Q_i)]$$

where $Q_i = c_i V_i$ is the total quantity of the ion in the inside compartment. Thus the internal specific activity increases in the way shown in Fig. 1.4(a) until, at infinitely large t, $S_i = S_o$. At the start

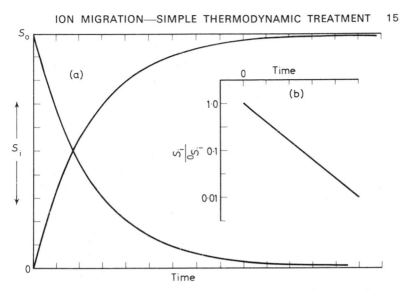

Fig. 1.4   (a) *Exponential increase or decrease of specific activity* (S_i) *in a single compartment, with time.* S_i *reaches* S_o *after equilibrium.* (b) *The specific activity as a proportion of that at the start of elution* ($S_i/{}^0S_i$) *plotted on a log scale against time*

of this process the rate of increase of S_i or of Y_i is linear and then, conveniently,

$$\phi = \frac{\Delta Y_i}{\Delta t} \cdot \frac{1}{S_o} \cdot \frac{1}{A} \tag{1.21}$$

If S_i is not negligible but comparable with S_o, then ϕ can still be obtained from

$$\phi = -\frac{2 . 203 \, Q_i \log_{10}(1 - S_i/S_o)}{t^* A}$$

where t^* is the time of the uptake experiment.

(b) For elution, $S_o = 0$ and $S_i = {}^0S_i$ at $t = 0$. Therefore

$$\frac{d Y_i}{dt} = -\phi_{io}^* A = -S_i \phi A$$

or

$$\frac{dS_i}{dt} = -\frac{S_i \phi A}{Q_i}$$

which, when integrated, gives

$$S_i = {}^0S_i \exp\left(-\phi At/Q_i\right)$$

t is now the time of elution. This equation is plotted as the second curve in Fig. 1.4(a). The same remarks apply to the initial part of the negative exponential decrease in S_i or Y_i. The radioactive appearing in the external solution during this time leads to an estimate of the flux through the relation

$$\phi = \frac{\Delta Y_o}{\Delta t} \cdot \frac{1}{S_i} \cdot \frac{1}{A} \qquad (1.22)$$

If there were a net flux across the surface, different equations would have to be used which took into account that Q_i was a function of time. However, if Q_i were sufficiently constant for short times, Eqs. (1.21) and (1.22) would lead to the influx and efflux, respectively.

Sometimes a useful description of the isotopic exchange across the surface can be given through the rate constant or some similar parameter that describes the exponential curves of Fig. 1.4(a).

A single parameter emerges when the log of S_i is plotted against time, as in Fig. 1.4(b), i.e. $\ln S_i = \ln {}^0S_i - \phi At/Q_i$. The slope of the straight line obtained is $-\phi A/Q_i$. $\phi A/Q_i$ is termed the rate constant k, of dimension time^{-1}. It can easily be verified that it is related to the 'half-time' for the exchange (the time for S_i to reach $\frac{1}{2}S_o$ (uptake) or for S_i to drop to $\frac{1}{2}{}^0S_i$ (elution)). In fact $t_{\frac{1}{2}} = 0.693/k$.

Plotting the data with a log scale for Y_i or S_i is a useful test for surface-controlled exchange.

1.8.2 Two compartments in series

Compartment 1 is a thin peripheral layer just inside the outer surface and the areas presented to compartments 0 and 2 are taken as equal. This model (Fig. 1.5) might be likened to a vacuolated plant cell. Restricting discussion to a steady state, the equal unidirectional fluxes at the outer boundary will be called ϕ_p (for plasmalemma) and at the inner ϕ_t (for tonoplast).

The relations between the radioactivity of the separate compartments (or of the compartments 1 and 2 together—the 'whole cell') and time are more complicated than those found for one compartment. However, if the rate constants of the two compartments are sufficiently different, certain parameters may be calculated from data taken from a log plot of Y_{total} against time. For a two-compartment model such a plot may resemble Fig. 1.6. Two rate constants k_L (for 'long' times) and k_S (for 'short') can be calculated, as well as Y_L and Y_S, from the analysis. These quantities are then

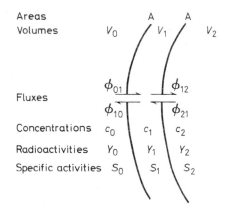

Fig. 1.5 *The quantities considered in relating radioactivity or specific activity to time when there are two series-connected compartments*

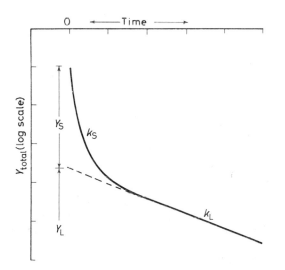

Fig. 1.6 *The total radioactivity (Y_{total}) plotted on a log scale against time of elution from a two-compartment system. Under favourable circumstances two rate constants k_S and k_L can be estimated, and corresponding radioactivities at the start of elution, Y_S and Y_L*

related to the fluxes ϕ_p and ϕ_t, and the constant quantities of substance in 1 and 2, Q_1 and Q_2, through the following relations for unit area (Pallaghy and Scott, 1969):

$$\phi_p = \frac{1}{S_o}\left(\frac{k_S Y_S}{1 - \exp k_S t^*} + \frac{k_L Y_L}{1 - \exp k_L t^*}\right) \tag{1.23a}$$

$$Q_1 = S_1 \phi_p^2 \bigg/ \left(\frac{k_S^2 Y_S}{1 - \exp k_S t^*} + \frac{k_L^2 Y_L}{1 - \exp k_L t^*}\right) \tag{1.23b}$$

$$\phi_t = Q_1\left(k_L + k_S - \frac{Q_1 k_L k_S}{\phi_p}\right) - \phi_p \tag{1.23c}$$

$$Q_2 = \phi_p \phi_t / k_S k_L Q_1 \tag{1.23d}$$

where t^* is the time of uptake. The relations are exact for the assumptions made, i.e. no net flux and perfect mixing in all spaces, 0, 1 and 2.

The differential equations appropriate to the two compartments are, for uptake,

$$\frac{dS_1}{dt} = \frac{\phi_{01}}{Q_1} S_o - \frac{\phi_{10} + \phi_{12}}{Q_1} S_1 + \frac{\phi_{21}}{Q_1} S_2$$

$$= \frac{\phi_p}{Q_1} S_o - \frac{\phi_p + \phi_t}{Q_1} S_1 + \frac{\phi_t}{Q_1} S_2$$

$$\frac{dS_2}{dt} = \frac{\phi_{12}}{Q_2} S_1 - \frac{\phi_{21}}{Q_2} S_2$$

$$= \frac{\phi_t}{Q_2} (S_1 - S_2)$$

When elution is considered, $S_o = 0$; otherwise the equations are as above. Analytical solution of these simultaneous equations is tedious. It has been found quick and convenient to solve for S_1/S_0, S_2/S_0 and Y_1, Y_2, $Y_1 + Y_2$ with a simple analogue computer. Figure 1.7 illustrates the rise and fall of fractional specific activities in the two phases during uptake and elution of radioactivity. The graphs show several features characteristic of the model of two series-connected compartments.

(a) Compartment 1, assumed to be small in capacity, reaches a relative specific activity somewhere between zero and 1 (in fact equal to $\phi_p/(\phi_p + \phi_t)$) and then climbs parallel with S_2.

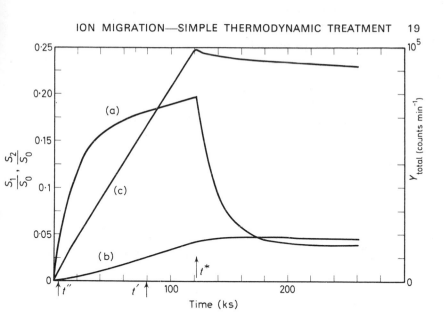

Fig. 1.7   *Solutions from an analogue computer of the differential equations for the specific activities of compartments 1 and 2 as functions of time. Curve (a) represents S_1 as a proportion of S_0. Curve (b) represents S_2 as a proportion of S_0. Curve (c) is total radioactivity in the compartments using an arbitrary value of 10^{12} C min^{-1} equiv.$^{-1}$ for S_0. The other values assumed were: $\phi_p = 10^{-12}$ equiv. cm^{-2} s^{-1}, $\phi_t = 5 \times 10^{-12}$ equiv. cm^{-2} s^{-1}, $Q_1 = 10^{-7}$ equiv. cm^{-2}, $Q_2 = 2 \times 10^{-6}$ equiv. cm^{-2}. At the time t^* shown by the arrow the effect is shown of suddenly reducing the specific activity outside to zero. This represents the elution of the compartments with inactive medium. The times t' and t'' are referred to in the text*

(b) There is a time lag before compartment 2 starts increasing in activity.

(c) When elution is started, in so far as $S_1 > S_2$ at the beginning of elution, radioactivity goes both from 1 to 2 and from 1 to 0. Compartment 2 increases in activity before falling. However, the total radioactivity declines with time, according to the sum of two negative exponentials, as already described.

When fluxes or quantities for the ion under investigation have been estimated from Eq. (1.23a–d), the computer solution, if these quantities are used, should confirm the shape of the elution curve. Alternatively, the experimental data can be fitted with fluxes ϕ_p and ϕ_t and quantities Q_1 and Q_2 by trial and error, which is a reasonable proposition with an analogue machine.

1.8.3 Short-cuts to the estimation of fluxes in two-compartment systems

Fluxes can be estimated approximately if the specific activity of the two compartments can be estimated separately. In some plant cells a physical separation can be made following a period in radioactive solution and the specific activity of 1 and 2 (cytoplasm and vacuole) estimated by measurement of radioactivity and by chemical analysis.

MacRobbie (1966b) has shown that at a time corresponding to t' in Fig. 1.7, when the specific activities of 1 and 2 are rising together,

$$\phi_t = Q_2 S_2 / t'(S_1 - S_2) \tag{1.24}$$

A second method takes advantage of the fact that at times near t'' in Fig. 1.7 $S_2 \ll S_1$, and the specific activity of 1 is rising with a time course given approximately by a simple exponential

$$S_1 Q_1 = \phi_{01} A[1 - \exp(-k_1 t)]/k_1 \tag{1.25}$$

where k_1 is the rate constant for the process of labelling compartment 1, and equals $A(\phi_{10} + \phi_{12})/Q_1$. Furthermore, for times up to t'', the total radioactivity of 1 and 2 combined rises linearly with time, and since $S_1 < S_0$,

$$Y_1 + Y_2 = \phi_{01} A . t \tag{1.26}$$

Therefore, the proportion of radioactivity in compartment 1 is

$$Y_1 / (Y_1 + Y_2) = \frac{1 - \exp(-k_1 t)}{k_1 t} \tag{1.27}$$

k_1 is estimated by a graphical method when the left-hand side of Eq. (1.27) and t are known. Next, Eq. (1.26) leads to ϕ_{01}, and, if Q_1 can be measured directly, $k_1 . Q_1$ gives $\phi_{10} + \phi_{12}$.

Whether or not these methods are practicable depends on whether the times t' and t'' are convenient in relation to the time taken to perform the separation of compartments.

2

Ion migration from the viewpoint of steady state thermodynamics

2.1 HISTORY

There are very cogent reasons for having to come to grips with a new kind of thermodynamics. Classical thermodynamics is restricted to reversible processes, or systems at equilibrium, and to closed systems. The very definition of the term 'equilibrium' is found in basic thermodynamic theory. Biological systems have few equilibria until they are dead, and are open systems. For a formal scheme unifying processes that are irreversible—diffusion is one—or systems that are in a steady state, we turn to a modern theory due mainly to Onsager. Treatments accessible to physicists date back only 15–20 years and applications to membranes, and to biological flow processes in particular, were made only about 10 years ago. Readers are referred to DeGroot and Mazur (1962) and to Katchalsky and Curran (1965). The latter book is specifically for biophysical applications.

2.2 FORCES AND FLOWS

There are many phenomena in nature in which a force causing a particular flow also results in an apparently unrelated flow. In the Peltier effect a flow of electric current caused by an e.m.f. (the force) is associated with a flow of heat. Semiconductor materials such as bismuth telluride can be used to cool a sector of the environment to below ambient temperature by the passage of direct current.

Onsager (1931) proposed that the flux of a component depends possibly on *all* the thermodynamic forces operating in the system, *in a linear way*. The justification for the linearity is found deep in the textbooks but is discussed qualitatively by Denbigh (1951). It holds only for processes not going 'too' fast, or not 'far' from equilibrium.*
Thus

$$\phi_1 = L_{11}X_1 + L_{12}X_2 + \cdots + L_{1n}X_n$$
$$\phi_2 = L_{21}X_1 + L_{22}X_2 + \cdots + L_{2n}X_n \qquad (2.1)$$
$$\vdots$$

In Chapter 1, considering *independent* fluxes, we wrote equations equivalent to

$$\phi_1 = L_{11}X_1, \quad \phi_2 = L_{22}X_2, \quad \ldots$$

ϕ_j and X_j in Eqs. (2.1) are called conjugate flows and forces, L_{ij} are called phenomenological coefficients, and Eqs. (2.1) are a set of phenomenological equations. By a rough sort of analogy with 'action and reaction are equal and opposite', an important reduction in the number of necessary coefficients comes about because of the reciprocal relations $L_{ij} = L_{ji}$, provided that the conjugate flows and forces are expressed in such a way that the rate of entropy production times temperature, and per unit volume, is given by the sum of the products of these flows and forces, i.e. $\Phi = \sum_j X_j\phi_j$, Further, since in irreversible processes the entropy production is always positive, it can be shown that $L_{ii}L_{jj} \geqslant L_{ij}^2$. Apart from these restrictions, the Onsager coefficients are independent; they have the meaning of generalised conductances, since they are in effect flow per unit force (cf. the permeabilities or mobilities discussed in Chapter 1).

An alternative way of writing phenomenological equations is to express the force on one sort of particle in terms of all the fluxes. Thus $X_1 = R_{11}\phi_1 + R_{12}\phi_2 + \cdots$, and, in general,

$$X_i = \sum_{j=1}^{n} R_{ij}\phi_j \qquad (2.2)$$

where the R_{ij} now have the meaning of a resistance coefficient—force per unit flow. Once again there is a set of reciprocal relationships $R_{ij} = R_{ji}$. There will be occasion to use both sets of equations involving L_{ij} or R_{ij}.

---

* Sometimes it is not clear what restrictions this causes, a difficulty that might be regarded as negligible compared with that of relating forces and flows in a biological system.

In a non-rigorous way this covers the important features of Onsager's equations. In dilute solutions the particles are so far apart on the average that the interaction is small, but as soon as concentrations of about $0 \cdot 25 – 0 \cdot 5$ M are reached, the cross-coefficient representing interaction between KCl and NaCl diffusing in water is about one-quarter of the magnitude of the straight coefficient (Fujita and Gosting, 1960).

It is time to look at some of the relevant phenomena in more detail. In particular, the phenomenological coefficients are related to combinations of the more familiar properties encountered in Chapter 1. Finally the phenomenological coefficients can be interpreted in terms of frictional interactions between particles and membranes, thus giving one possible physical interpretation of the coefficients.

2.3 INTERACTIONS

2.3.1 A system with three flows

It is proposed to confine attention to the flows and forces operating in the relatively simple system: uni-univalent electrolyte solution/membrane/uni-univalent electrolyte solution.

The electrolyte solution has three main components if ion-pairs are neglected. These components are cations, anions and water molecules. When the membrane material is included, there are four possible interactions: ion–ion, ion–water, ion–membrane and water–membrane.

It is necessary to consider the fluxes of each of the three components in terms of the forces operating on all of them. Subscripts 1, 2 and 3 refer to cations, anions and water:

$$\phi_1 = L_{11}X_1 + L_{12}X_2 + L_{13}X_3$$
$$\phi_2 = L_{21}X_1 + L_{22}X_2 + L_{23}X_3 \tag{2.3}$$
$$\phi_3 = L_{31}X_1 + L_{32}X_2 + L_{33}X_3$$

For the purpose of this exercise, following a treatment of Kedem and Katchalsky (1963), the forces to be used are the 'reduced forces':

$$X_1 = \Delta\bar{\mu}_1, \quad X_2 = \Delta\bar{\mu}_2, \quad X_3 = \Delta\bar{\mu}_3$$

The electrochemical potentials for ions have already been defined.

The difference in chemical potential of water is

$$\Delta\mu_3 = \Delta\mu_w = \overline{V}_w(\Delta P - \Delta\pi_s)$$

where $\Delta\pi_s$ is the osmotic potential corresponding to the difference in concentration Δc_s. (The subscripts 'w' and 's' represent 'water' and 'solute', respectively.)

2.3.2 Transposition of forces and flows

It is somewhat more convenient to transpose Eqs. (2.3) to equations relating more easily observed flows, and more easily measured driving forces. It is quite permissible to choose other conjugate forces and flows provided that their products lead to the same entropy dissipation rate.

Starting with

$$\Phi = \phi_1\Delta\bar{\mu}_1 + \phi_2\Delta\bar{\mu}_2 + \phi_w\Delta\mu_w \qquad (2.4)$$

it is noted that $\Delta\mu_s = \Delta\bar{\mu}_1 + \Delta\bar{\mu}_2$, where $\Delta\mu_s$ is chemical potential difference of the ionizing solute. $J = F(\phi_1 - \phi_2)$ gives the density of electric current through the membrane; then define an e.m.f. acting across the membrane as being given by the difference in electrochemical potential difference for the anions, i.e. $\Delta V = \Delta\bar{\mu}_2/F$, which is equivalent to the difference between the p.d. indicated by salt bridges with reversible half-cells ($\Delta\psi$, or ψ_m in Chapter 1) and the Nernst potential for species 2. Substituting for ϕ_1, ϕ_2, $\Delta\bar{\mu}_1$, $\Delta\bar{\mu}_2$ in terms of the fluxes of electricity and solute (Kedem and Katchalsky, 1963) the dissipation function now becomes

$$\Phi = \phi_s\Delta\mu_s + \phi_w\Delta\mu_w + J\Delta V$$

$$= \phi_w\overline{V}_w(\Delta P - \Delta\pi_s) + \phi_s\overline{V}_s\Delta P + \phi_s(\Delta\pi_s/\bar{c}_s) + J\Delta V \qquad (2.5)$$

$\bar{c}_s$ is an average concentration within the membrane defined by $\bar{c}_s = \Delta\pi_s/\Delta\mu_s = \Delta\pi_s/(RT\Delta \ln a_s)$.

When the membrane is not ideally semi-permeable, ϕ_s is finite and any observed volume change on either side *is not due to* ϕ_w alone. What is observed is a *volume* flow given by

$$\phi_v = \overline{V}_w\phi_w + \overline{V}_s\phi_s \qquad (2.6)$$

With this change, and re-arrangement,

$$\Phi = \phi_v(\Delta P - \Delta\pi_s) + \phi_s(\Delta\pi_s/\bar{c}_s)(1 + n_s) + J\Delta V \qquad (2.7)$$

$n_s = \overline{V}_w\bar{c}_s$ is the approximate mole fraction of solute. $1 + n_s$ is about unity for practical purposes (a molal solution has one molecule of solute to every 55·5 of water).

Thus, the new conjugate flows and forces are

Volume flow: pressure-osmotic potential difference
Solute flow: chemical potential difference
Electric current flow: electromotive force = electrochemical potential difference for the anions

The new phenomenological equations are (with different L_{ij} since the dimensions of the flows and forces are different even though the dimensions of their products are still entropy . temperature . time^{-1} but per unit area):

$$\phi_v = L_{11}(\Delta P - \Delta \pi_s) + L_{12}(\Delta \pi_s/\bar{c}_s) + L_{13}\Delta V$$
$$\phi_s = L_{21}(\Delta P - \Delta \pi_s) + L_{22}(\Delta \pi_s/\bar{c}_s) + L_{23}\Delta V \qquad (2.8)$$
$$J = L_{31}(\Delta P - \Delta \pi_s) + L_{32}(\Delta \pi_s/\bar{c}_s) + L_{33}\Delta V$$

with $L_{ij} = L_{ji}$ as before.

2.3.3 Practical coefficients

The relation between the phenomenological coefficients and the many observed experimental coefficients can now be quickly written down—the patient reader is rewarded.

First, reverting to the classical situation, where cross-coefficients are assumed zero we would write:

$$L_{11} = \phi_v/(\Delta P - \Delta \pi_s)_{L_{ij} = 0(i \neq j)}$$

is the hydraulic conductivity ($cm^3 \, cm^{-2} \, s^{-1} \, atm^{-1} = cm \, s^{-1} \, atm^{-1}$).

$$L_{22} = \phi_s/(\Delta \pi_s/\bar{c}_s)_{L_{ij} = 0(i \neq j)}$$

is the solute permeability.

$$L_{33} = (J/\Delta V)_{L_{ij} = 0(i \neq j)}$$

is the electric conductance (mho cm^{-2}).

In the more complex but more realistic situation where the L_{ij} are not zero, the straight coefficients are related to fluxes per unit force only by making various forces or flows zero in the imagined measurement.

If both sides of the membrane are accessible any two of the conjugate forces of Eqs. (2.8) could be made zero by the following means.

Conditions of the forces	Means used to bring about these conditions
(a) $\Delta P - \Delta \pi_s = 0$ $\Delta \pi_s = 0$ therefore $\Delta P = 0$	No solute gradient and the pressure is equalised from outside.
$\Delta V \neq 0$	Applied e.m.f. $= \Delta V$. From (2.8) $L_{13} = \phi_v/\Delta V$ is the electro-osmotic volume flow; $L_{23} = \phi_s/\Delta V$; $L_{33} = J/\Delta V$ is the electrical conductance.
(b) $\Delta \pi_s = \Delta V = 0$	No solute gradient and an e.m.f. is applied to keep $$\Delta \psi = -\frac{RT}{F} \ln (a_2^o/a_2^\delta)$$ whence $L_{11} = \phi_v/\Delta P$ is the filtration co-efficient (hydraulic conductivity); $L_{21} = \phi_s/\Delta P$; $L_{31} = J/\Delta P$ is the streaming current per unit pressure difference.
(c) $\Delta P - \Delta \pi_s = 0$ $\Delta V = 0$	To accomplish this one might apply a pressure on the concentrated side to stop volume flow. However, although $\phi_v \rightarrow 0$, there will be finite ϕ_s and ϕ_w such that $\phi_s/\overline{V}_s = -\phi_w/\overline{V}_w$. In general, there will be a streaming potential associated with these fluxes and a current would be applied to bring the membrane potential back to $\Delta \psi$. Such an applied current would change ΔP through the cross-coefficient L_{31} but this might be regarded as a second-order effect.

Assuming that (c) can be done:

$$L_{12} = \phi_v/(\Delta \pi_s/\bar{c}_s)$$
$$L_{22} = \phi_s/(\Delta \pi_s/\bar{c}_s) \text{ is the solute permeability}$$
$$L_{32} = J/(\Delta \pi_s/\bar{c}_s) \text{ is the permeation current}$$

Before leaving this set of coefficients, it must be pointed out that certain *combinations* of them are identical with other well-known and often-measured parameters. Under conditions (a) $\phi_v/J = L_{13}/L_{33}$ is the electro-osmotic permeability (sometimes the symbol β is used for this) and $\phi_s/J = L_{23}/L_{33} = t^+/F$, where t^+ is the transport number for the cations. Under conditions (b) and (c) similar pairs of ratios can be defined. There are certain difficulties about making pairs of forces vanish, as seen particularly in (c) above. Two other sorts of restrictions, one force and one flow are zero, or two flows are zero, lead to other relations between flows and forces which are represented by single phenomenological coefficients.

Details of these procedures should be sought in Staverman's article (1952) or that of Kedem and Katchalsky (1963).

2.4 FRICTIONAL COEFFICIENTS

2.4.1 Definitions

When a force is applied to a particle such as an ion, the ion quickly reaches a constant average velocity. Hence, it must be supposed that an equal and opposite equivalent 'force' analogous to friction on the macroscopic scale operates to keep the acceleration zero. Furthermore, since a property such as 'mobility' or velocity per unit electric force is constant for varied forces, the 'frictional force' opposing the otherwise certain acceleration must be proportional to velocity. On the sub-microscopic scale the 'friction' is merely repeated collisions with other particles of the solution or membrane.

The frictional force on 1 mol of particles is now defined by the product of a frictional coefficient and the relative velocity between the particles considered, e.g. species i has a force

$$X_{ij} = -f_{ij}v_{ij} = -f_{ij}(v_i - v_j) \qquad (2.9)$$

on it due to species j, where f_{ij} is the frictional coefficient (force on 1 mol* of i by all the species j for unit relative velocity: the units are dyne mol^{-1} cm^{-1} s or J s mol^{-1} cm^{-2}) and v_{ij} is the mean relative velocity of particles i and j; v_i and v_j are velocities with reference to a stationary object such as the membrane. X_{ij} is shown as a negative quantity for positive relative velocity because it is a vector in the opposite direction to that of the driving force.

* Other frictional coefficients have been defined which represent the mutual interaction between 1 mol of i and 1 mol of j. These are 'reduced friction coefficients'.

2.4.2 Addition of frictional forces

In the steady state the driving force is balanced by the sum of the frictions of all the species encountered during migrations, i.e.

$$X_i = -\operatorname{grad} \bar{\mu}_j = -\sum_{j(\neq i)} X_{ij}$$

$$= \sum_{j(\neq i)} f_{ij}(v_i - v_j) \tag{2.10}$$

Returning to the model system used in Eqs. (2.3) and dealt with by Speigler (1958), we would have for the two ion species (1) and (2), water (3) and the membrane material (4) the following frictional coefficients between ions and water *within the membrane*: $f_{12}, f_{13}, f_{14}, f_{23}, f_{24}, f_{34}$. Thus the driving force on the cations is balanced such that

$$X_1 = f_{12}(v_1 - v_2) + f_{13}(v_1 - v_3) + f_{14}v_1 \tag{2.11a}$$

Similarly,

$$X_2 = f_{21}(v_2 - v_1) + f_{23}(v_2 - v_3) + f_{24}v_1 \tag{2.11b}$$

The velocities, and later, concentrations refer to particles within the membrane. Because of the particular definition of the f_{ij} relating to 1 mol of i and an indefinite amount of j, the equilibrium of forces for the water molecules must be written for the *total* forces acting:

$$X_3 + X_{31} + X_{32} + X_{34} = 0$$

i.e.

$$c_3X_3 + c_1X_{13} + c_2X_{23} + c_3X_{34} = 0$$

whence,

$$X_3 = -[(c_1/c_3)f_{13}(v_1 - v_3) + (c_2/c_3)f_{23}(v - v_3) - f_{34}v_3] \tag{2.11c}$$

It is to be noted that through Newton's law of action and reaction

$$c_1f_{13} = c_3f_{31} \tag{2.12}$$

From the Eqs. (2.11a–2.11c) v_1, v_2 and v_3 may be obtained in terms of the frictional coefficients. Then, since

$$\phi_j = v_jc_j \tag{2.13}$$

the fluxes can be written in the form of Eqs. (2.3) with the phenomenological coefficients appearing as complicated functions of the cs and fs.

A useful simplification (but one that may not be as widely applicable as is assumed) is to suppose that in a negatively charged membrane the concentration of mobile anions might be small compared with the concentration of counterions. Hence, f_{12} might be neglected. This was done by Spiegler (1958). The consequence of so doing is mentioned in Chapter 3 in the discussion of results for an ion exchange membrane investigated by Mackay and Meares (1959).

The phenomenological coefficients are given at the end of the chapter in terms of f_{ij} and other quantities. Before leaving the subject, we outline the procedure for obtaining the frictional coefficients in terms of relatively easily measurable quantities.

2.4.3 Measurements to enable calculation of f

It is supposed that the experimental situation is one of the simpler ones used in Eqs. (2.3) above to show the relations between Onsager coefficients and commonly measured transport coefficients.

Experiment (i)
Set $\Delta P = \Delta \pi_s = 0$; $J = 0$. That is, there exist equal concentrations of electrolyte on each side of the membrane. Then it is supposed that there are two isotopic forms of the cations, which, starting separately, are allowed to mix by penetrating the membrane. Under these conditions $X_2 = X_3 = 0$.

If the solutions are perfectly stirred on each side, the rate of passage of isotope is related to the coefficient of self-diffusion for the cations within the membrane—D_1. It may be shown that

$$D_1 = RT/(f_{13} + f_{14}) \qquad (2.14)$$

if f_{12} is neglected in comparison with the other frictions; and

$$D_2 = RT/(f_{23} + f_{24}) \qquad (2.15)$$

D_1 and D_2 can be measured experimentally, and with the aid of three further measurements, outlined below, all five f_{ij} can be calculated.

Experiment (ii)
Set $\Delta P = \Delta \pi_s = 0$. Apply an e.m.f. from outside the membrane and measure the electro-osmotic water flow. Strictly, what is observed is *volume* flow, because we cannot stop a small volume change due to the fluxes of anions and cations. However, since these are in opposite directions and the partial molar volumes of the ions are somewhat similar, the volume flow closely approximates the water flow.

Spiegler calls the electro-osmotic flow coefficient Ω. It has the units mol $(cm^2 \ s)^{-1}$. $(V \ cm^{-1})^{-1}$. It was seen in Section 2.3 that an electro-osmotic volume flow was given by $L_{13} = \phi_v/\Delta V$. This is a volume flow per unit e.m.f., not per unit potential gradient. Also, the phenomenological coefficients of Sub-Section 2.3.3 are different from the present ones, since the forces are now $-\text{grad } \bar{\mu}_1$, etc., and not the 'reduced forces' ΔP, $\Delta \pi_s$, etc.

With unit potential gradient across the membrane, and with equal concentrations on each side, the forces X_1, X_2 and X_3 are simply expressed:

$$X_1 = -\text{grad } \bar{\mu}_1 = -\frac{\partial}{\partial x}(\mu_1^0 + RT \ln a_1 + F\psi)$$

$$= F \quad \text{if} \quad \frac{\partial \psi}{\partial x} = -1$$

$$X_2 = -F, \quad X_3 = 0$$

therefore

$$\Omega = (\phi_3)_{(\frac{\partial \psi}{\partial x}) = 1} = (L_{31} - L_{32})F \qquad (2.16)$$

with a more complicated expression when the Ls are replaced with the correct functions of c_i, f_{ij} (see Section 2.7).

Experiment (iii)
As for (*ii*), set $\Delta P = \Delta \pi_s = 0$. Measure the electric current density for unit potential gradient. This equals the membrane conductivity σ. Therefore

$$\sigma = F(\phi_1 - \phi_2)_{(\frac{\partial \psi}{\partial x}) = 1} = F^2(L_{11} - 2L_{12} + L_{22}) \qquad (2.17)$$

Experiment (iv)
The proportion of the electric current carried, say by the cation, is determined with radioactive tracers under the same conditions as (*ii*) and (*iii*):

$$t^+ = \phi_1/(\phi_1 - \phi_2) = \frac{L_{11} - L_{12}}{L_{11} - 2L_{12} + L_{22}} \qquad (2.18)$$

Spiegler points out that rather accurate measurement of these quantities is necessary before the frictional coefficients can be calculated meaningfully.

A further simplification is possible when the membrane is a cation exchanger and the external concentrations are kept low compared with the concentration of the immobile groups A_- in the membrane. Then $c_2 \ll c_1$ and f_{23}, f_{24} can be neglected.

Calculations of frictional coefficients in real membranes are referred to in the next chapter.

2.5 FRICTIONAL COEFFICIENTS AND PHENOMENOLOGICAL RESISTANCE COEFFICIENTS

It has already been seen how the 'conductance' type of Onsager coefficients (L_{ij}) can be written in terms of the frictional coefficients. This formulation is particularly simple for the 'resistance' type of Onsager coefficient. Assume the co-ion concentration in the membrane to be negligible. A comparison between Eqs. (2.19) and (2.20) then gives the required identities:

$$X_1 = - \text{grad } \bar{\mu}_1 = f_{13}(v_1 - v_3) + f_{12}(v_1 - v_2) + f_{14}v_1$$

$$X_2 = - \text{grad } \bar{\mu}_2 = f_{23}(v_2 - v_3) + f_{21}(v_2 - v_1) + f_{24}v_2 \qquad (2.19)$$

$$X_3 = - \text{grad } \bar{\mu}_3 = f_{31}(v_3 - v_1) + f_{32}(v_3 - v_2) + f_{34}v_3$$

which are identical with

$$\begin{aligned} X_1 &= (f_{12} + f_{14})v_1 - f_{12}v_2 - f_{13}v_3 \\ &= [(f_{12} + f_{13} + f_{14})\phi_1/c_i] - (f_{12}\phi_2/c_2) - (f_{13}\phi_3/c_3) \\ X_2 &= (f_{21} + f_{23} + f_{24})v_2 - f_{21}v_1 - f_{23}v_3 \\ &= (-f_{21}\phi_1/c_1) + [(f_{21} + f_{23} + f_{24})\phi_2/c_2] - (f_{23}\phi_3/c_3) \\ X_3 &= (f_{31} + f_{32} + f_{34})v_3 - f_{32}v_2 - f_{31}v_1 \\ &= (-f_{31}\phi_1/c_1) - (f_{32}\phi_2/c_2) + [(f_{31} + f_{32} + f_{34})\phi_3/c_3] \end{aligned} \qquad (2.20)$$

whence

$$R_{11} = (f_{12} + f_{13} + f_{14})/c_1, \quad R_{12} = - f_{12}/c_2, \quad R_{13} = - f_{13}/c_3$$

$$R_{21} = - f_{21}/c_1, \quad R_{22} = (f_{21} + f_{23} + f_{24})/c_2, \quad R_{23} = - f_{23}/c_3$$

$$R_{31} = - f_{31}/c_1, \quad R_{32} = - f_{32}/c_2, \quad R_{33} = (f_{31} + f_{32} + f_{34})/c_3$$

where c_1, c_2, c_3 are local concentrations at a given plane x. Thus the frictional forces are functions of x, and the velocities therefore are also functions of x (going from o to δ) but the product of velocity and concentration is a constant (equal to the flux) in the steady state.

2.6 EFFECT OF FRICTIONAL INTERACTION ON FLUX RATIOS

If we use the second form of the phenomenological equations, a linear relation between forces and flows is assumed, thus:

$$X_i = \sum_{j=1}^{n} R_{ij}\phi_j$$

If we focus attention on two isotopes '1' and '2' of a monovalent ion species,

$$X_1 = R_{11}\phi_1 + \sum_{j(\neq 1)} R_{1j}\phi_j = - \text{grad } \bar{\mu}_1$$

$$X_2 = R_{22}\phi_2 + \sum_{j(\neq 2)} R_{2j}\phi_j = - \text{grad } \bar{\mu}_2$$

(2.21)

On rearranging Eq. (2.21),

$$\phi_1 = -\frac{1}{R_{11}}\left(\frac{d\bar{\mu}_1}{dx} + \sum_{j(\neq 1)} R_{1j}\phi_j\right)$$

$$\phi_2 = -\frac{1}{R_{22}}\left(\frac{d\bar{\mu}_2}{dx} + \sum_{j(\neq 2)} R_{2j}\phi_j\right)$$

(2.22)

The direct coefficients R_{11} and R_{22} are put inversely proportional to the local concentration of 1 and 2 in the membrane, so that $R_{11} = F_1/c_1$, $R_{22} = F_2/c_2$ (compare Section 2.5); and since 1 and 2 are isotopes, $F_1 = F_2$, $R_{1j} = R_{2j}$ $(j \neq 1, 2)$.

Putting $\bar{\mu}_1 = P\bar{V}_1 + RT\ln a_1 + F\psi + \mu_1^0$, and making a further assumption that there is no interaction between isotopes in the membrane, i.e. $R_{12} = 0$, Hoshiko and Lindley (1964) showed that the flux ratio is

$$\phi_1/\phi_2 = -(a^o/a^\delta)\exp\left[-\left(\bar{V}\,\Delta P + F\,\Delta\psi + \int_o^\delta \sum_{j(\neq 1, 2)} R_{1j}\phi_j\,dx\right)/RT\right]$$

This equation should be compared with the simpler one that was obtained without consideration of interactions. In a steady state, if there are any net fluxes besides those of the isotopes, the flux ratio is *not* obtained from the activity ratio and p.d. across the membrane but is affected by all other fluxes. In natural systems, as pointed out by Kedem (1961), these other fluxes may include flows of metabolites or metabolic products as well as the more obvious flows of ions and water. The drag between these fluxes and the primary flux (1 or 2) is sometimes referred to as 'entrainment'.

Meares (1959) also developed a flux ratio equation in terms of frictional coefficients in much the same way as did Hoshiko and Lindley. Both Kedem and Essig (1965) and Coster and George (1968) have adopted a more general approach to the effects of interaction on the flux ratio, and on the crossover potential, at which influx = efflux; this potential is not now exactly equal to the Nernst potential. In these treatments isotope interaction is specifically allowed for.

The difficulty in using these general equations lies in the number of the unknown resistance coefficients. In some simple situations it is possible to evaluate approximately the importance of the interaction terms (Chapter 3).

2.7 APPENDIX

In Sub-section 2.4.2 the procedure was outlined for obtaining phenomenological coefficients in terms of frictional forces. The relations between the L_{ij} and f_{ij} are finally established through Eqs. (2.11) and (2.13), neglecting f_{12}.

Then

$$L_{11} = \frac{c_1[(c_1 f_{13} + c_3 f_{34})(f_{23} + f_{24}) + c_2 f_{23} f_{24}]}{\substack{c_1 f_{12} f_{14}(f_{23} + f_{24}) + c_2 f_{23} f_{24}(f_{13} + f_{14}) \\ + c_3 f_{34}(f_{13} + f_{14})(f_{23} + f_{24})}} \tag{A.1}$$

$$L_{22} = \frac{c_2[(c_2 f_{23} + x_3 f_{34})(f_{13} + f_{14}) + c_1 f_{13} f_{14}]}{D} \tag{A.2}$$

where Eq. (A.2) has the same denominator, D, as (A.1);

$$L_{33} = \frac{c_3^2(f_{13} + f_{14})(f_{23} + f_{24})}{D} \tag{A.3}$$

$$L_{12} = L_{21} = \frac{c_1 c_3 f_{13} f_{23}}{D} \tag{A.4}$$

$$L_{23} = L_{32} = \frac{c_2 c_3 f_{23}(f_{13} + f_{14})}{D} \tag{A.5}$$

$$L_{13} = L_{31} = \frac{c_1 c_3 f_{13}(f_{23} + f_{24})}{D} \tag{A.6}$$

The set of L_{ij} from Eqs. (A.1–A.6) are then used in Eqs. (2.3) with the appropriate conservative forces $d\bar{\mu}_j/dx$ (Sub-section 2.4.3).

3

Experiments with non-living membranes

3.1 ADVANTAGES OF ARTIFICIAL MEMBRANES

The biologist is fortunate to be able to draw upon a store of knowledge built up from experiments with non-living membranes. Compared with biological membranes, non-living ones may offer several simplifications. These simplifications come about because of homogeneity of membrane material, relative permanence (existence over a wider range of environments) and the opportunity to make changes and measurements on both sides of the membrane. Thus it is possible to measure a number of transport properties on the same membrane.

One of the more complete studies of ion exchange membranes has been made by Mackay, Meares and Ussing (references below). The purpose of this chapter is to draw attention to the properties that have been studied in ion exchange and other non-living membranes, including the recently rediscovered 'bimolecular layer' membranes. In all this we shall be particularly concerned with those aspects of relevance to biological membranes.

3.2 ION EXCHANGE MEMBRANES

3.2.1 Diffusion coefficients and ion activities

Mackay and Meares (1959) measured the electrical conductivity and electro-osmotic permeability of a resin membrane, Permutit Zeo-Karb 315, a cation exchanger with a capacity of about 0·5 mequiv. per cubic centimetre of imbibed water. From these and measurements made by Meares (1959) it was possible to calculate the self-diffusion coefficients for Na^+ and Cl^- within the membrane. The object was to test for electrostatic interaction between the counterions and the resin fixed ions, and for increases in viscosity of the water very near the fixed ions. These were possible contributing factors to an unexpectedly low diffusion coefficient of the counterions previously reported by other investigators.

Eventually Mackay and Meares were able to estimate frictional coefficients for the Zeo-Karb membrane on the basis of the Spiegler model (see Chapter 2).

The diffusion coefficients for Na^+ and Cl^- are given in Table 3.1. D_{Na} increased greatly with external concentration. This corresponded

Table 3.1   SELF-DIFFUSION COEFFICIENTS (cm^2 s^{-1} $\times$ 10^6) IN A CATION EXCHANGE MEMBRANE (FROM MACKAY AND MEARES, 1959)

[NaCl] (mol l^{-1})	D_{Na}	D_{Cl}
0·01	2·33	7·50
0·02	2·97	7·46
0·05	3·51	7·42
0·10	3·72	7·37
0·50	4·75	7·23
1·00	4·70	7·08

to an increasing number of mobile co-ions in the resin and an increasing number of Na^+ ions migrating away from the sites of electrostatic interaction or increased solvent viscosity. D_{Cl} was relatively constant, understandably so, since the anions are electrostatically repelled from the fixed charges. D_{Cl} was less than the value in free solution (about $1·5 \times 10^{-5}$) owing to tortuosity in the paths followed in the resin. The even lower values of D_{Na} at the lower concentrations were consistent with the modified conditions for diffusion near the fixed ions, mentioned above. It was shown that ion-pair formation or 'binding' was not involved because the electro-osmotic coefficient $(J_v/\Delta E)_{\Delta P=0}$ was greater with the dilute external solutions, where D_{Na} is smaller. The increased concentration of electric charge near the resin as c_o increases led to less interaction between Na^+ and H_2O. In addition, Cl^- in increasing concentration in the matrix pores tended to cause electro-osmotic volume flow in the opposite direction from that of Na^+.

Mackie and Meares (1955) pointed out that the theory of concentrated electrolytes does not apply to the ions sorbed into an ion exchange resin. The activity coefficient of the counterions decreases with decreasing concentration, the opposite to what is observed in aqueous solutions.

Kobatake *et al.* (1965) found that the correct activity for the counterions in a highly charged membrane is given by the concentration of co-ions, i.e. for a cation exchanger

$$a^+ = c^- = a^- \tag{3.1}$$

That is, if we look on the resin cations as being composed of two sorts, those paired with the resin anions and those with the co-ions, the activity coefficient of the cations of the first sort is very low.

3.2.2   Frictional coefficients

It was seen in Chapter 2 that Spiegler's treatment gave expressions for the frictional coefficients in terms of diffusion coefficients, concentrations, etc. (Eqs. 2.14–2.19). For dilute solutions, where f_{12} (representing the interaction between counterions and co-ions in the membrane) can be neglected, measurement of D_{Na}, D_{Cl}, t_{Na}, membrane conductance and electro-osmotic permeability enables calculation of the f_{ij}. Mackay and Meares (1959) calculated the values given in Table 3.2 for these coefficients, in Js cm^{-2} mol^{-1}. Recall that 1 stands for Na$^+$, 2 for Cl$^-$, 3 for H$_2$O and 4 for membrane matrix.

Table 3.2

f_{13}	f_{14}	f_{23}	f_{24}	f_{34}
4.93×10^8	2.13×10^8	3.32×10^8	0.02×10^8	0.05×10^8
f_{13}^0 1.86×10^8		f_{23}^0 1.22×10^8		

In addition, the calculated frictional coefficients for diffusion in an open aqueous medium (superscript 0) are given for comparison. It is seen that for the counterions the friction due to the membrane material is a significant part of the total opposition to migration, and that due to water is much greater than when the ions are diffusing in water in the absence of a membrane. Part of this increase is due to differences in the mole fraction of water and to tortuosity.

Further information comes from a comparison of some of the fs at different external concentrations (see Table 3.3). It can now be appreciated that the variation in D_{Na} as a function of c_o, referred to in Table 3.1, stems from changes in f_{13} and not so much from f_{14}. Hence, the suggestion of increased viscosity of the solution near the fixed charges is entirely reasonable.

Table 3.3

$c_o(\text{mol}^{-1})$	f_{13}	f_{14} (Js cm^{-2} mol^{-1} $\times$ 10^8)	f_{23}
0·01	8·10	2·53	0·06
0·02	6·00	2·34	0·40
0·05	4·94	2·12	3·48
0·10	4·63	2·03	2·75

Spiegler (1958) calculated the frictional coefficients for a membrane of sodium polymethacrylate resin from data of Despic and Hills (1956). It is interesting to compare these with the results of Mackay and Meares in Table 3.2:

f_{13}	f_{14}	f_{34}	f_{13}^0
$2·59 \times 10^8$	$6·4 \times 10^8$	$0·05 \times 10^8$	$2·39 \times 10^8$

Once again the friction between water and membrane material, per mole of water and unit relative velocity, is small compared with that between sodium ions and water or membrane, on the same basis.

3.2.3 Flux ratios

Meares and Ussing (1959) set out to test the flux-ratio equation (Chapter 2), including in their investigation the effect of mutual drag or friction between the flux of the substance considered and all the other substances, particularly water. If the flux of co-ions through the membrane is low, the main 'drag term' is due to the net flux of water. As well as an expression for the flux ratio under these conditions, the authors also derived expressions for the net flux and for the expected membrane p.d.

The fluxes were measured with the aid of radioactive tracers for Na^+ and Cl^-. P.d.s were measured for various concentrations of NaCl on each side of a Zeo-Karb 315 membrane and corrected for liquid junction p.d.s between the calomel half-cells and the NaCl solutions.

The final expression for flux ratio is of interest, as it contains a single term expressing interaction in place of the integral in the equation of Hoshiko and Lindley (Chapter 2):

$$\ln(\overrightarrow{\phi}/\overleftarrow{\phi}) = \ln(c^o/c^\delta) + \ln(\gamma^o/\gamma^\delta) + \frac{zF\,\Delta\psi}{RT} + \frac{\overline{V}\,\Delta P}{RT} + \frac{\sigma\delta}{D} \qquad (3.2)$$

where most of the symbols have already been defined but in addition σ is the mean rate of flow of all components in the x-direction; most of the volume flow is due to water. D is the self-diffusion coefficient (within the membrane) of the ion of which the fluxes are to be measured.

The relative importance of the several terms in Eq. (3.2) is seen from Table 3.4, which compares observed and calculated flux

Table 3.4

c^o $\quad c^\delta$ (mol l^{-1})		$\ln(c^o/c^\delta)$	$\ln(\gamma^o/\gamma^\delta)$	$zF\Delta\psi/RT$	$\dfrac{\sigma\delta}{D}$	$\ln(\overrightarrow{\phi}/\overleftarrow{\phi})_{calc}$	$\ln(\overrightarrow{\phi}/\overleftarrow{\phi})_{obs}$
1·0	0·1	2·303	−0·097	−0·727	−0·236	1·243	1·335
0·5	0·1	1·609	−0·097	−0·716	−0·191	0·605	0·737
1·0	0·5	0·693	0·000	−0·062	−0·051	0·580	0·542
0·1	0·1 + HCl	0·000	0·000	+0·327	+0·185	0·512	0·560

ratios of Na$^+$. ΔP was zero. Curiously, better agreement is obtained by omitting the activity coefficient term, but there is no justification for this.

The importance of the term containing the effect of solvent friction is obvious. In other words, the simple flux-ratio equation of Chapter 1 is inadequate for non-living membranes, let alone biological ones.

Further data were obtained with the same resin but with equal concentrations on each side and with a p.d. applied to vary the flux ratio. Meares (1959) used these results to test predictions for the flux ratio based on Spiegler's model. In this model, it will be recalled, there is a balance between frictional forces and driving forces on the ion species considered. For the simplified situation where $c^o = c^\delta$ and $\gamma^o = \gamma^\delta$

$$\ln(\overrightarrow{\phi}/\overleftarrow{\phi}) = (F\,\Delta\psi + f_{13}v_3\delta)/RT \qquad (3.3)$$

where v_3 is the solvent velocity, a known function of c_1, c_2, c_3 and the frictional coefficients.

Since the concentrations in the resin membrane and the frictional coefficients were known from previous considerations (Tables

3.2, 3.3), it was possible again to compare observed flux ratios and those calculated with the aid of Eq. 3.3. Some of the comparisons for chloride and sodium ion fluxes are included in Table 3.5. The agreement is seen to be fairly good for sodium fluxes. By contrast,

Table 3.5

Ext. conc. (mol l⁻¹)	p.d. (mV)	$\ln(\vec{\phi}/\overleftarrow{\phi})_{calc}$	$\ln(\vec{\phi}/\overleftarrow{\phi})_{obs}$
		(Fluxes of Na⁺)	
0·01	−5·3	0·41	0·45
0·01	−10·5	0·82	0·89
0·02	−10·1	0·68	0·75
0·02	−20·5	1·38	1·30
0·05	−23·0	1·43	1·47
0·05	−32·0	2·00	1·81
		(Fluxes of Cl⁻)	
0·05	8·4	0·19	0·04
0·05	16·2	0·36	0·48

the agreement with data on chloride fluxes is not at all good. This was attributed to the omission in the derivation of frictional coefficients and flux ratios of terms involving the frictional coefficient f_{21}. Although co-ions are in the minority within the membrane, the effect of numerous counterions upon them might be appreciable.

3.3 CELLULOSE MEMBRANES

Ginzburg and Katchalsky (1963) used the thermodynamics of the steady state and considerations of frictional forces, now familiar to us, to obtain expressions for the hydraulic permeability, reflection coefficient and solute permeability in terms of the frictional coefficients. Although they are for non-ionic solutes and cellulose membranes (made from, for instance, dialysis tubing), the results of these calculations are included in this chapter for comparison with the ion–water, ion–membrane and water–membrane frictions already tabulated. Subscript s is used below for solute and 3 and 4 are used for water and membrane as before (Table 3.6). We note some of the same features that were apparent in the permeation of ion exchange membranes by ions and water. These are (a) friction between water and solute is greater than that between solute and membrane; (b) the coefficient representing friction between water

Table 3.6 f_{ij} in J s mol^{-1} cm^{-2} × 10^8

Membrane	Solute		f_{s3}	f_{s4}	f_{34}
Visking dialysis tubing	Urea	0·5M	6·6	0·65	0·083
	Glucose 0·05M		18·9	2·3	0·085
	Sucrose 0·025M		32·5	6·5	0·085
Dupont wet gel	Urea		2·8	0·046	0·017
	Glucose		7·8	0·30	0·017
	Sucrose		11·2	0·66	0·017

and membrane is again two orders of magnitude smaller than the other coefficients; and (c) f_{s3} and f_{s4} increase as the size of the penetrating molecule increases.

3.4 VERY THIN MEMBRANES

There has been a revival of interest in the properties of artificially made, thin, lipid membranes. Since these can be made only a few molecules in thickness, they are of great interest in relation to natural membranes, which are probably a bimolecular leaflet of lipids with associated proteins (Chapter 4).

Dean, Curtis and Cole (1940) seem to have been the first to prepare a membrane of 'molecular thickness'. It was formed of lecithin and egg albumin. The electric resistance, capacitance and phase angle were measured. More recently Mueller et al. (1963) have prepared membranes ∼70Å thick from extracts of brain lipids; and Hanai, Haydon and Taylor (1964), from lecithin with up to 50% n-decane. Bilayers of rhodopsin were studied by Takaga, Azuma and Kishimoto (1965).

Mueller and Rudin (1967) reported that thin membranes of sphingomyelin could be made to behave like relaxation oscillators and to produce a large potential difference when separating solutions of 0·1 N KCl and 0·1 N NaCl if an extract called 'excitation inducing material' (EIM) were added. Before the addition the membrane was electrically stable and the p.d. was very small. The induced phenomena resembled those observed in living cell membranes. Other investigators have been concerned with the permeability of thin membranes to water and a comparison between the results obtained when that permeability is measured in two different ways. The water permeability measured for an osmotic or pressure gradient, P_{os}, and that measured with the aid of radioactive water, P_d, in the absence of an osmotic or pressure gradient are sometimes found to be different. When $P_{os} > P_d$, bulk flow through pores in the membrane is deduced. A theory involving these permeabilities, the effective pore diameter and other factors is given by Kedem and Katchalsky (1961).

Table 3.7 contains a summary of some of the physical properties of artificial, bimolecular membranes. They have a high electric resistance (with the exception of rhodopsin), in the range 10^6–10^9 $\Omega\,cm^2$ and a capacitance of about 0·5 $\mu F\,cm^{-2}$. When unstirred layers are thoroughly accounted for (Cass and Finkelstein, 1967), P_{os} and P_d become nearly equal. In the other experiments P_d may have been underestimated owing to this factor (see Dainty, 1963), but even so a real difference between P_d and P_{os} is claimed.

Certain classes of antibiotics have been discovered to cause spectacular changes in the resting conductance of ultra-thin membranes. Valinomycin, a macrocyclic depsipeptide, causes an increase in conductance, particularly when KCl solutions bathe the membrane. Valinomycin is regarded as causing a change to specific permeability to K^+ (Lev and Buzhinski, 1967; Andreoli, Tieffenberg and Tosteson, 1967). Other substances such as the gramicidins cause a change towards cation selectivity.

Polyene antibiotics such as nystatin penetrate ultra-thin membranes, provided that they are of mixed (phospholipid and cholesterol) composition and cause massive increases in anion permeability (van Zutphen, van Deenan and Kinsky, 1966; Finkelstein and Cass, 1968).

A close study of the interactions between membranes and such permeability modifiers may well lead to more precise concepts of the molecular structure and function of natural membranes.

3.5 APPLICATIONS TO BIOLOGICAL MEMBRANES

The relevance to biological membranes should now be apparent. Thorough studies such as the ones dealing with ion exchange membranes which have been described have enabled many conclusions to be drawn about the physical basis of ion permeation. If equally sophisticated studies could be made of natural membranes, we might decide some of the following questions.

(a) Do ions permeate by diffusing with the usual mobility (or a reduced one) through a few large pores?

Table 3.7

Membrane material	Resistance (Ωcm^2)	Capacitance ($\mu F\ cm^{-2}$)	Water permeability (cm s^{-1}) P_{os}	P_d	Ref.
Phosphatidyl choline, cholesterol and n-decane	10^9	0·52	$1·9 \times 10^{-3}$	$2·2 \times 10^{-4}$	Hanai, Haydon and Redwood (1966)
Phosphatidyl choline, n-tetradecane	—	—	$2-9 \times 10^{-3}$	4×10^{-4}	Thompson and Huang (1966)
	$10^4-5 \times 10^5$	—	—	—	Takaga, Azuma and Kishimoto (1965)
Phospholipid	10^7	—	10^{-3}	10^{-3}	Cass and Finkelstein (1967)
Phospholipid + EIM	$1-2 \times 10^4$	—	10^{-3}	10^{-3}	Cass and Finkelstein (1967)
Sphingomyelin	10^6	—	—	—	Mueller and Rudin (1967)
Sphingomyelin + EIM	2×10^5	—	—	—	—
Cholesterol + phospholipid	10^8	0·4	—	—	Andreoli, Bangham and Tosteson (1967)

(b) Do they diffuse through a larger number of smaller pores?

(c) What is the extent of interaction between ions and water in the membrane? If zero, then presumably ions dissolve in the membrane material individually. If so, what is their concentration?

(d) What is the extent of interaction between one-way fluxes of the same ion, between fluxes of cations of various sorts, and between ions and metabolites?

Some progress has been made with some of these problems and they will be referred to in the appropriate chapters.

It is time now to look at models of biological membranes as described by various visionaries.

4

Visualisation of the structure of biological membranes

This chapter is intended to be a brief summary of what is surmised about the structure of biological membranes. The word 'visualisation' is appropriate when we remember that these structures are 'submicroscopic' in thickness. Most electron micrographs of membranes so far have been of dead preparations; recently, more sophisticated preparations are claimed to be more likely to be artifact-free. Moor and Mühlethaler (1963) used deep-frozen cells, fractured the surface of the cell with a freezing ultramicrotome, and took a carbon replica of the part of the surface. If cells such as yeast were thawed following the deep-freeze, they survived.

Our mental concept of biological membranes crystallised with the advent of Davson's and Danielli's model. This was at first a bimolecular layer of lipid. Later it was thought that denatured protein must be bonded to each side (Danielli and Davson, 1952). The physical properties of such a model are matched in some respects by those of cell membranes (see Chapter 3, and Briggs, Hope and Robertson, 1961). There are, however, several objections to this simple model.

(a) It would lack enzymic activity in the denatured or spread protein. At this stage there seemed room for no more than 10–20Å width of protein on each side.

(b) Moderate-sized molecules could apparently not permeate except by dissolving in the lipid phase.

(c) Small particles such as ions and water would also have to permeate by dissolving in the lipid. Virtual pores or slits due to random motion of the molecules of the membranes seemed somewhat unlikely, owing to its 'solid' nature.

In other words, the requirement that the structure be in a condensed phase to give permanence goes with so many van der Waals' bonds that the probability of pores opening spontaneously seemed low.

Stein and Danielli (1956) therefore proposed that there are permanent, protein-lined pores or openings, big enough to allow some types of molecules to enter but infrequent enough to account for the low observed permeability to such molecules.

The resistance of lipid bilayers is 10^6–10^9 Ω cm^2 (Chapter 3) but less when proteins are 'added'. The resistance of cell membranes is usually 10^3–10^4 Ω cm^2 (Chapter 7). The difference suggests that natural membranes are not structurally similar to the artificial membranes. These latter, from their minimum thickness and other considerations, are probably arrays of molecules with long chains normal to the surface and with polar groups facing outwards towards the aqueous phases, much as proposed by Danielli and Davson (1952). The way in which added protein or EIM affects structure as it lowers the resistance is simply not known at present.

Recent studies with the electron microscope (Moor and Muhlethaler, 1963) appeared to reveal clusters of globular material on the outer surface of membranes. These globules, 50–150Å in diameter, were interpreted as globular protein. Frey-Wyssling (personal communication) believes the new evidence from electron microscopy to be consistent with membranes having a basic bimolecular layer of lipids with globular protein added. Thus objection (a) above would be removed.

Other workers, concentrating on the structure of lipids in solution, propose that natural membranes could equally well be composed of micelles of lipid. When these are packed in a hexagonal array, there are holes with a maximum opening of about 4Å (Lucy, 1964). The stability of such a membrane is in some doubt compared with that of the Davson–Danielli model, which has the possibility of many more van der Waals' bonds to keep it together. Nevertheless, Paganelli and Solomon (1957) showed that we may need to think of red blood cell membranes as having pores of an 'operational' radius 3·5Å if their behaviour towards the permeation of water is to be accounted for. Perhaps the lipid micelle concept of cell membranes would remove objection (c) above.

Branton (1966) has questioned the interpretation of the Zurich school that the globules observed are on the surface of the membrane facing an aqueous phase. His studies seem to show that when the

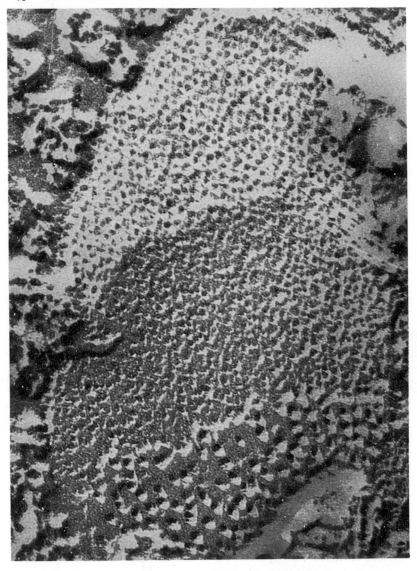

Fig. 4.1 *The inner and outer surfaces of two neighbouring stroma thylakoids in a chloroplast from spinach. Magnification:* × 171 000.(*From Mühlethaler, Moor and Szarkowski, 1965. Reproduced by kind permission of the authors and of* Planta. *Photomicrograph supplied by Drs A. Frey-Wyssling and K. Mühlethaler*)

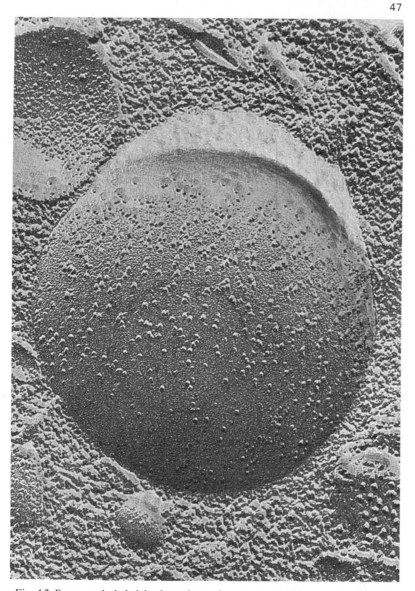

Fig. 4.2 *Freeze-etched thylakoid membrane from a spinach chloroplast, covered with 120 Å particles. Magnification:* × *ca.* 112 000. (*From Mühlethaler, Moor and Szarkowski,* 1965. *Reproduced by kind permission of the authors and of* Planta. *Photomicrograph supplied by Drs A. Frey-Wyssling and K. Mühlethaler*)

freezing ultra-microtome fractures the preparation, the membrane splits along the middle. The subsequent etching and replica-taking then reveals the structure in the median plane of the membrane. The globules so revealed may be either protein or lipid.

Figures 4.1 and 4.2 illustrate the surface of the membranes of stroma and grana in chloroplasts (thylakoid membranes), showing clearly the hemispherical globules, about 120Å in diameter.

5

Membrane potentials and relative ion permeabilities

5.1 INTRODUCTION

Manifestations of electricity in living things have fascinated scientists since Galvani's day. The electric voltage found across the surface of most, if not all, living cells is interesting in its own right. As an important part of the total force acting to move ions, it deserves, and has received, study in a large number of plant and animal cells.

It seems almost certain that the p.d.s in living cells are diffusion potentials of one sort or another. In these systems, discussed for simple situations in Chapter 1, the p.d. is caused by a minute separation of charges on ions, at one or more planes in the system. A small minority opinion regards the p.d. as being a redox potential as though electrolytic contact were being made with 'electrodes' in cells equivalent to the noble metal electrodes used in normal redox measurements *in vitro*. Although scientists' votes do not establish the truth of majority opinion, it still seems that the evidence for the ionic theory is overwhelming. This is not to say that redox reactions are not coupled to membrane p.d.s through the cell's metabolism. Readers interested in the redox hypothesis for cellular potentials are referred to articles by Lund and co-workers (Lund *et al.*, 1947).

5.2 PERMEABILITY DEDUCED FROM MEMBRANE POTENTIALS

It is proposed in this chapter to see, by use of some examples of simpler systems, such as single giant axons, muscle fibres, internodal cells of Characean species and marine coenocytes, how well the ionic theory accounts for the observations.

5.2.1 *Sepia* **axons**

With *Sepia* (cuttlefish) axons in sea-water containing 10·4 mN K$^+$, the mean p.d. with 0·2 mM dinitrophenol (DNP) in the medium was 63 mV (Hodgkin and Keynes, 1955 b). The inside of the cell was negative to the bathing medium. The p.d. could be altered by changing K_o, keeping K_o + Na_o constant at 490 mN. The treatment with DNP was designed to eliminate an active influx of potassium which may have confused estimates of 'potassium conductance' (see Chapter 7).

Figure 5.1 shows the relation between the p.d. and K_o. The mean axoplasm concentrations (not activities) were 270 mequiv. K$^+$ per litre axoplasm and 58 of Na$^+$. As a first approximation it might be thought that the axons were permeable solely to K$^+$ so that

$$\psi_m = 58 \log_{10}(K_o/270) \tag{5.1}$$

This corresponds to Eq. (1.5) for the Nernst potential. It is apparent that the equation corresponds with the observations only at the higher concentrations and then only moderately well. A big improvement is obtained in the closeness of fit if the effect of probable permeation of sodium ions is allowed for in the equations for ψ_m:

$$\psi_m = 58 \log_{10} \frac{P_K K_o + P_{Na} Na_o}{P_K K_i + P_{Na} Na_i} \tag{5.2}$$

which corresponds to Eq. (1.12). In the full curve of Fig. 5.1, $P_{Na}/P_K = \alpha = 0·03$. K_i has been put at 310 mequiv. per litre axoplasm water instead of 270 mequiv. per litre axoplasm.

Thus to a second approximation the axolemma is permeable to K$^+$ and Na$^+$ in a constant ratio of about 30:1 over a wide range of K_o and ψ_m. The effect of sodium is pronounced when K_o is low.

Refinements could be made to the theoretical considerations (by use of activity coefficients and by examining the effect of permeability to other ions and the effect of potential-dependent permeability) but the main conclusion would stand, that potassium permeability dominates. For example, Strickholm and Wallin (1967) made a careful study of the permeability coefficients for K$^+$, Na$^+$ and Cl$^-$ needed to describe the p.d. in giant axons of crayfish (*Procambarus clarkii*) as K_o was varied. P_{Cl}/P_K was 0·13 when ψ_m was -83 mV (K_o, 5·4 mM) but increased to 0·85 at -53 mV (K_o, 25 mM).

A further test of the ionic hypothesis was made possible when it was learnt that the axolemma (membrane) of *Loligo* (squid) axons was left relatively unharmed after the extrusion of the axoplasm by a miniature garden-roller followed by perfusion with solutions of K_2SO_4, etc. (Baker, Hodgkin and Shaw, 1961). When the potassium

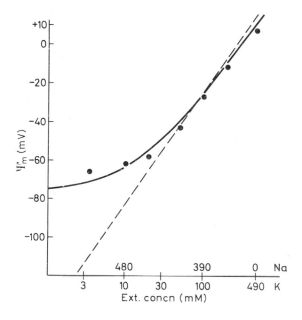

Fig. 5.1 *Data from Table 1 of Hodgkin and Keynes* (1955 b) *showing the way the intracellular p.d. in DNP-treated axons from* Sepia officinalis *changed with the concentration of potassium in the external solution. The sum of* K_o + Na_o *was kept constant at* 490 mequiv. 1^{-1}. *The circles are experimental points; the dashed line is the relation between* ψ_m *and* K_o *calculated from Eq.* (5.1), *the full line, as calculated from Eq.* (5.2)

concentration of the perfused solution was varied, the p.d. between inside and outside also changed. However, the effect of K_i decreased between 150 and 600 mN, possibly because P_K decreased. Nevertheless the theory is better than qualitative and also predicted the level of the peak of the action potential as Na_i was varied, with the permeability ratio P_{Na}/P_K then about 10. The phenomenon of membrane excitability is beyond the scope of this book, although it is clearly related to it. *The Sherrington Lectures VII* (Hodgkin, 1964) are a valuable account of some of the classical work.

5.2.2 Single muscle fibres

Similar experiments were done by Hodgkin and Horowicz (1959 a) with single muscle fibres dissected from frogs (*Rana temporaria*). In these cells, which are quite permeable to both K^+ and Cl^-, when K^+ is simply changed for Na^+, or Cl^- for $SO_4^=$ outside, there is net loss or gain of KCl and gain or loss of water. The system behaves as a Donnan system that comes to equilibrium at a rate determined by the sarcolemma (membrane) permeabilities to K^+ and Cl^-, and possibly by diffusion rates within the fibre protoplasm. The influence of internal diffusion on ionic relations will be discussed later.

In the muscle fibres, when $K_o \times Cl_o$ was kept constant but K_o and Cl_o varied reciprocally (neutrality was maintained with Na^+ and $SO_4^=$), net fluxes of salt or water were not expected. The reason for this lies in the nature of the Donnan equlibrium, at which

$$\psi_K = 58 \log_{10}(K_o/K_i)$$

and

$$\psi_{Cl} = 58 \log_{10}(Cl_i/Cl_o)$$

At equilibrium $\psi_m = \psi_K = \psi_{Cl}$; thus, if equilibrium is to be maintained and merely ψ_m altered, then

$$K_o/K_i = Cl_i/Cl_o$$

or
$$K_o Cl_o = K_i Cl_i = \text{const.}$$

Figure 5.2 shows that the p.d. changed in the expected way and corresponded to that calculated from the measured K_i and Cl_i, namely 140 mequiv. K^+ per kilogramme fibre H_2O and 2·14 of Cl^-.

In the absence of Cl^- and with $SO_4^=$ the anion, when K_o was changed, the p.d. changed almost exactly according to

$$\psi_m = 58 \log_{10} \frac{K_o + 0·01\ Na_o}{140}$$

which showed that the sarcolemma had a slight permeability to Na^+. When fibres were in Ringer's solution with K_o 2·5 mN and Cl_o 120 mN, P_K/P_{Cl} was about 0·5. This ratio did not stay constant in other solutions.

5.2.3 *Chara* and *Nitella*

Experiments with these cells date back a great many years and it is possible that they were the subject of the first experiments employing glass microelectrodes (Umrath, 1930), although these electrodes were not the micron-sized ones subsequently developed by Graham and Gerard (1946).

Plant cells are more complicated than animal cells in that there are more identifiable phases. However, the fact that the vacuoles of

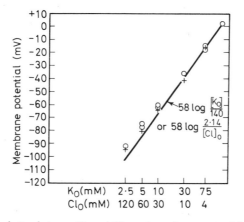

Fig. 5.2   *The relation between* K_o *and* Cl_o, *and membrane potential in single muscle fibres (Fig. 4 from Hodgkin and Horowicz, 1959 a). In these experiments* $K_o \times Cl_o$ *was kept constant at 300 mM². The crosses refer to membrane p.d.s 10–60 min after changing a solution, and circles, 20–60 s after a sudden change. (Reproduced by kind permission of the authors and of* The Journal of Physiology)

these particular plant cells contain only crystallites is a simplification for electrical measurements. Owing to the presence of a cell wall that is an inhomogeneous cation exchange phase (Dainty and Hope, 1959, 1961), the results of experiments in which the p.d. is measured while K_o and Na_o are changed are harder to interpret.

When the external medium or the pond water of their origin contains calcium and relatively low concentrations of K^+ and Na^+, the cell walls are largely populated with divalent counterions. Possibly the plasmalemma also has charges that are paired with Ca^{++}. When, now, K_o is changed for Na_o ($K_o + Na_o$ being kept constant), there is often little change in the p.d. measured between the vacuole and outside. Presumably the insensitivity to K_o/Na_o changes is due to the extreme slowness of change of the concentration of these ions just outside the plasmalemma. It was seen in Chapter 3 from studies of ion exchange membranes that the diffusion coefficient for Na^+ was low within these membranes when the ionic strength outside was low. The exchange of Ca^{++} in the cell walls for Na^+ in the medium was particularly slow in *Chara* (Dainty and Hope, 1959). In any case, when calcium ions are exchanged from the cell wall by prolonged soaking in solutions of a uni-univalent electrolyte, the plasmalemma becomes a '$K_o + \alpha Na_o$' electrode rather like the axolemma, with $\alpha (= P_{Na}/P_K)$ constant (*Chara*: Hope and Walker, 1961) or increasing somewhat when K_o is made very small (*Nitella*: Spanswick, Stolarek and Williams, 1967). α was 0·1 in *Chara australis** and 0·1–0·3 in *Nitella translucens*.

The most complete study of concentrations of the main ions in the cytoplasm and vacuole and of the p.d.s across the plasmalemma and tonoplast is that by Spanswick, Stolarek and Williams (1967). There are several other species that have been worked on intensively, but this will serve to summarise the 'steady state' situation in non-growing cells (Table 5.1).

The cell wall. This phase is not expected to distinguish between K^+ and Na^+ to a first approximation, and is observed not to change p.d. appreciably when K_o is changed with $K_o + Na_o$ kept constant (Spanswick, Stolarek and Williams, 1967). Hence, changes between the cytoplasm and outside reflect exactly the changes across the plasmalemma. We should, however, look briefly at the meaning of the 'cell wall potential' given prominence by Nagai and Kishimoto (1964). When a microelectrode is placed very close to or within the cell wall phase, there is a quasi-equilibrium; the following concentration cell yields a p.d.:

calomel half-cell : 3 N KCl (reference electrode) : artificial pond water (APW) : cell wall : 3 N KCl (micro-electrode) : calomel half-cell

If more were known about the diffusion of KCl within the cell wall, the p.d. could be predicted. Assuming only Donnan potentials, if A, the effective concentration of indiffusible ions in the wall, is 600 mN (Dainty and Hope, 1961), the p.d. would be about − 100 mV, when the external medium is APW. If the wall comes to equilibrium during measurements of intracellular (not intra-wall) p.d., simple thermodynamic considerations show that the same p.d. would be observed whether a cell wall were present or not, provided that the permeability to anions is negligible (Hope and Walker, 1961). The level of efflux of chloride shows that this is almost true $(P_{Cl}/P_K \sim 10^{-3})$ and therefore conclusions about the plasmalemma deduced from

---

* The species name for what was previously *Chara australis* was changed in 1968 to *C. corallina*, thus lessening national pride in what was probably the species of *Chara* with the largest cells, including Texan ones (up to 2 mm in diameter or up to 25 cm long).

Table 5.1 CONCENTRATIONS (mequiv. 1^{-1}) AND P.D.S (mV) IN CELLS OF *Nitella translucens*

ψ_{vo}	ψ_{co}	ψ_{vc}	K_v	K_c	Na_v	Na_c	Cl_v	Cl_c	Ref.
−121	−138	−17	75	119	65	14	—	—	Spanswick and Williams (1964)
−118	−137	−19	—	—	—	—	160	65	Spanswick and Williams (1964)
−126	−141	−15	69	93	73	37	—	—	Spanswick, Stolarek and Williams (1967)

The external medium was APW: 0·1 mN KCl, 1·0 mN NaCl and 0·2 mN CaCl₂ for the first line; Ca₀ was zero in the other experiments. v is for vacuole, c for cytoplasm.

studies of p.d.s are not affected by the cell wall phase. If the cell wall is not at thermodynamic equilibrium, one has to be exceedingly cautious about conclusions regarding possible electrochemical equilibrium for particular ions, based on Nernst's equation, as we shall see below.

5.2.4 Marine algae

High permeability to K^+ relative to Na^+ and Cl^- is found in some marine algae such as *Halicystis ovalis* and in several *Griffithsia* species. However, the plasmalemma of cells of *Chaetomorpha darwinii* responds in its p.d. to changes in Cl_o, as well as to changes in K_o or Na_o. *Valoniopsis* and *Boergesenia* resemble *Chaetomorpha* in this respect. The p.d. of the vacuole is small, being from -10 to $+10$ mV with respect to sea-water. This p.d. consists of a negative step across the plasmalemma and a positive p.d. across the tonoplast, which two steps largely cancel out.

In *Griffithsia*, Findlay, Hope and Williams (1969) estimated α to be $0 \cdot 002 – 0 \cdot 006$, this genus having the most potassium-selective natural membrane known. In all the marine algae studied, the cytoplasm is approximately from -50 to -90 mV with respect to sea-water. The relative permeabilities and cytoplasmic activities that might account for these observations have not been determined except for *Griffithsia*.

5.3 THE PHYSICAL BASIS OF SELECTIVITY TOWARDS IONS

5.3.1 Membrane selectivity

Changes in potential between the inside and outside of a cell occur when the concentration of ions is changed outside (Section 5.2 above). There seems good reason to suppose that this is connected with the cell membrane and its relative permeability to ions, although some of the observed effects would be obtained at the boundary between a Donnan phase and its bathing medium, even if the boundary were easily permeated by ions. Thus qualitatively the same changes in p.d. might be obtained following an increase in concentration outside (a) a membrane selectively permeable to cations (e.g. having negatively charged permeable areas) and (b) a negatively charged 'open' phase such as gelatin or pectin. Both would become more negative on the side made more concentrated.

We now have to enquire what property of ions or membranes leads to graded selectivity between cations. For example, both $P_K > P_{Na}$ and $P_{Na} < P_K$ are observed at cell surfaces; discrimination in favour of K^+ seems the more common. A sieving effect in which the smaller hydrated ions are allowed through would mean that potassium ions would always be preferred to sodium. A theory outlined by Eisenman (1960, 1962) shows that selectivity in membranes or in a macroscopic phase should be based on the following factors.

(a) The probability of an ion leaving an aqueous solution to exchange with a counterion in another phase depends on the change in free energy in the exchange.

(b) There will be differences in the free energy change according to the extent of change in the hydration of the ions in becoming adsorbed and desorbed.

(c) The electrostatic energy of interaction between the fixed negative ions and the adsorbed counterions will depend on both the fixed ions (their effective radius) and the counterions (their new hydrated size).

When all these factors are taken into account, it is found that various ion exchange materials, such as the newly developed cation responsive glasses, may exhibit preferences towards adsorbing cations in the two extreme orders

$$Cs > Rb > K > Na > Li$$

$$Li > Na > K > Rb > Cs$$

or in a number of other, intermediate patterns.

The anionic field strength is the most important factor determining the sequence of specificity, and the extent of hydration in the ion exchange material has more effect on the magnitude of the preference. That is, P_i/P_j depends on the extent to which the ion exchanger is hydrated but whether $P_i >, < $ or $= P_j$ depends on the nature of the anion and neighbouring atoms. Figure 5.3 shows plots of $\Delta F_{ij}^{7,6}$ against r_-, from Eisenman (1962). $\Delta F_{ij}^{7,6}$ is the calculated change in free energy for the exchange of 1 mol of i at a certain molality in the exchanger (7) for 1 mol of j at infinite dilution in the surrounding aqueous solution (6). r_- is the effective radius of the exchanger anions and partly determines the electrostatic energy of the bond formed with cations. When ΔF_{ij} is negative, j is preferred to i. In Fig. 5.3 i is always Cs^+.

Eisenman (1963) has assembled many data from biological

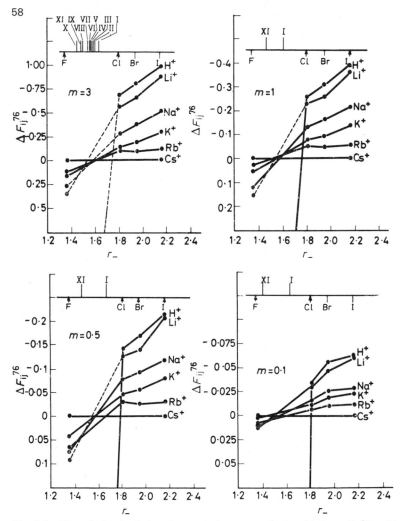

Fig. 5.3   *The calculated relative changes in free energy for ions i (always* Cs^+*) and j* (Rb^+, K^+, Na^+, Li^+, H^+*) in the transition from states 7 to 6, where 7 refers to a solution phase, and 6 to a hydrated ion exchange phase, are plotted against the effective radius of the anionic group in the ion exchanger* (r_-). *The calculations have been performed for four different assumed hydrations in the ion exchange phase, namely* 0·1, 0·5, 1 *and* 3 *molal. The Roman numerals refer to specificity orders, e.g.* I *is* $Li^+ > Na^+ > K^+$ $Rb^+ > Cs^+$, *in which the ion exchanger would select cations in numbers decreasing from* Li^+ *to* Cs^+ *if presented with equimolar activities in the adjacent solution. The anions* F^-, Cl^-, Br^- *and* I^- *were used as representative anions with a convenient spread of* r_-. *(From Eisenman, 1962. Reproduced by kind permission of the author and of the Rockefeller Institute Press, publishers of* Biophysical Journal*)*

experiments to compare with the theory. Generalisations can be made along the following lines.

(a) Selectivity towards cations estimated from resting potential and conductance and from resting fluxes corresponds to the region of low anionic field strength (the right-hand sides of the graphs of Fig. 5.3). The selectivity order spreads about series IV, which is K > Rb > Cs > Na > Li.

(b) Selectivity exhibited during excitation and by the outside of frog skin corresponds to a high anionic field strength and a sequence: Na > Li > (K, Rb, Cs).

It is to be noted that coulombic forces are overwhelmingly the main influence in ion adsorption when monovalent ions are considered. Further discussion of selectivity, including anion, and divalent cation selectivity, is to be found in an authoritative review by Diamond and Wright (1969).

5.3.2   Cytoplasmic selectivity

Sodium ions are found to be the minority of cations in cytoplasm, and potassium ions the majority, in many instances. This has been attributed to the action of an outwardly directed sodium pump (see further Chapters 6 and 9). Ling (1965, 1966) and others have maintained that the cytoplasmic ion population is the result of preferential adsorption of K^+ at fixed negative charges. The considerations of Sub-section 5.3.1 have indicated that such preference is theoretically possible. However, it is possible to show on simple thermodynamic grounds that the hypothesis of preferential adsorption of K^+ is not enough to account for the distribution of ions between the vacuole and medium of certain plant cells (Chapter 6). Evidence discussed in Chapter 7 also leaves little doubt that membranes control permeation rates in many instances.

5.3.3   The state of potassium in cytoplasm

It has been stressed above that, even in situations where potassium ions appear to be 'preferentially adsorbed', electrostatic forces form the normal bond between K^+ and the adsorption sites. That K^+ under these conditions is readily exchangeable, mobile and 'active' is indicated by two lines of evidence.

(1) The diffusion coefficient for K^+ in squid axoplasm is not much less than in aqueous solution, according to experiments made by Hodgkin and Keynes (1953). In these experiments the radio-activity from K-42 that had exchanged for axoplasmic K^+ at a restricted area on the surface was traced as it spread out along the interior of the axon. The redistribution, both with and without an applied electric gradient, was consistent with $D_K \simeq 1\cdot3 \times 10^{-5}$ cm^2 s^{-1} (for aqueous solutions $D_{KCl} \simeq 1\cdot5 \times 10^{-5}$ at 0·5 M and 18°C). As an estimated 90% of the axoplasmic potassium is exchangeable, there is nothing 'specially' mobile about the radioactive potassium introduced into the axon, as claimed by Troshin (1960).

(2) The activity coefficient of both K^+ and Na^+ within squid axoplasm and muscle fibres has been estimated by Hinke (1961) and Lev (1964) by means of cation-selective microelectrodes. The values of potassium and sodium activity and of the activity co-efficients are given in Table 5.2. Although the activity coefficient

Table 5.2   MEAN CONCENTRATIONS, ACTIVITIES AND ACTIVITY COEFFICIENTS FOR K^+ AND Na^+

j		c_j(mol 1^{-1})	a_j(mol 1^{-1})	γ_j	γ_{KCl}
		Axoplasm of *Loligo* in sea-water (Hinke, 1961)			
K^+	—	—	0·203	0·605	0·680
Na^+	—	—	0·037	—*	—
		Frog muscle fibres (Lev, 1964)			
K^+	A	0·13	0·098	0·77	0·75 (0·125 M)
	B	0·12	0·095	0·77	—
Na^+	A	0·029	0·0055	0·19	—
	B	0·028	0·0053	0·19	—

* 24% of the sodium possibly 'bound'.
A and B refer to values using microelectrodes with different selectivities towards K^+ compared with Na^+.

of potassium ions is high, that of sodium is surprisingly low. Cope (1967) reached the same conclusion about sodium through a study of the nuclear magnetic resonance signal from the sodium in muscle and other tissue.

Vorobiev (1967) made measurements in cells of *Chara* and *Griffithsia* using glass microelectrodes with the tips filled with material responsive mainly to potassium activity ($K_{NaK} \simeq 4$). In the cytoplasm of *Chara*, which was constantly streaming past the elec-trode tip, the potassium activity was about 110 mN.

These considerations lead one to reject for the present the idea that K^+ fits snugly into a lattice of cytoplasmic fixed changes and neighbouring ordered water molecules (Ling 1965), and in which it has a reduced mobility or activity. Sodium ions present more of a mystery.

There are some uncertainties in using microelectrodes of any sort in a phase as complicated as living cytoplasm and the conclusions must be provisional. It is probably realistic to believe that the ion activities found by the glass microelectrode method relate to the average activity in the material in contact with the glass. This region is claimed to be damaged (Ling, 1966).

5.4 CONCLUSIONS

An electric potential difference is commonly observed between the inside and outside of cells. In a 'normal' medium such as blood plasma the inside of an animal cell is electrically negative. Plant cells are more complicated. The p.d. between the vacuole and the external medium may be either positive or negative and is made up of p.d.s across the plasmalemma and across the tonoplast. The cytoplasm seems, in general, to be negative to the medium, corresponding approximately to the ratio of activity of potassium ions in the cytoplasm to that in the medium.

When the concentrations outside are changed, there is usually an immediate response in the p.d. Cells are normally depolarised by an increase in external potassium. The detailed way in which the p.d. changes with K_o ($K_o + Na_o$ being constant) is often well described by an equation that includes K_o and a fraction α of Na_o. α is the ratio of the permeability of the outer membrane for Na^+ to that for K^+; it is ~ 0.01 in several animal systems, ~ 0.1 in some Characean species and as small as 0.002 in a marine alga. Membranes or surfaces where the selectivity is in favour of sodium ions are rare. One example is the outer side of frog skin.

The selectivity displayed is probably a property of the outer membrane, in which ions have rather different mobilities and solubilities compared with aqueous solutions. The activity of potassium ions within cytoplasm appears to be comparable to that which they would have in an aqueous solution with the same concentration, but the activity of sodium ions appears inexplicably low.

6

Active and passive transport

6.1 THE NERNST POTENTIAL

The previous chapter showed that many cell membranes are permeable to potassium ions and to a lesser extent to sodium ions, and that some membranes are permeable to chloride ions as well, or instead. Also, large concentration gradients are observed across cell membranes. The question might be asked whether, given enough time, the solutions on each side of cell membranes come to an equilibrium. Large concentration gradients may be associated with a p.d. of the appropriate sign and magnitude and yet the system may be at equilibrium in the thermodynamic sense.

This approach is naive but not so naive as the idea (now history) that the finding of a higher concentration on the inside of a biological membrane than in the medium is evidence of 'active accumulation' of those ions.

In Chapter 1 the activity ratio of ions at equilibrium was shown to be associated with an equilibrium potential, the Nernst potential:

$$\psi_j = (RT/z_j F) \ln (a_j^o/a_j^\delta)$$

In many of the isolated, non-growing Characean cells the net flux of K^+, Na^+ and Cl^- may be very small under constant conditions. Finite permeability of these cells to the ions has been confirmed through measurements of ion fluxes (see Fig. 8.4), so that a tentative application of the Nernst criterion is warranted.

6.2 NERNST POTENTIALS FOR IONS IN *Nitella*

We have suitable data in Table 5.1 for calculating Nernst potentials, but the internal concentrations must be *corrected for activity*, which is appropriate for Eq. (1.5). The activity coefficient is taken (without much justification for the cytoplasm) as that for 160 mN KCl in both the cytoplasm and vacuole. This coefficient is 0·75 (Robinson and Stokes, 1955).

Thus we have the Nernst potentials given in Table 6.1. Several conclusions could be drawn from this table.

Table 6.1

	At the plasmalemma		At the tonoplast	
	A	B	A	B
ψ_{obs}	−138	−141	+17	+15
ψ_K	−171	−167	+12	+ 8
ψ_{Na}	− 84	− 59	−39	−17

Reference A is to Spanswick and Williams (1964); Reference B to Spanswick, Stolarek and Williams (1967).

(a) At the plasmalemma $\psi_K < \psi_{obs}$; therefore the activity of K^+ in the cytoplasm is too high to be an equilibrium value. Either the Nernst p.d. has been incorrectly estimated, or the net flux was not zero, or forces other than the 'physical' or 'passive' ones have acted on potassium ions to bring about the observed distribution across the plasmalemma. This discrepancy between ψ_K and ψ_{obs} led to the conclusion that some of the K^+ influx is active transport (MacRobbie 1962; Spanswick and Williams, 1964).

(b) At the plasmalemma $\psi_{Na} > \psi_{obs}$; therefore by similar reasoning there must be a component of active transport in the efflux of Na^+, so that the steady state activity is lower than the equilibrium activity for these ions.

(c) Chloride. In Table 5.1 the value for the concentration of chloride in the cytoplasm is probably much too high (Bradley and Williams, 1967; Coster and Hope, 1968). For the present, considering the chloride activity ratio between vacuole and outside, $\psi_{Cl} = +114$ mV and $\psi_{obs} = -118$ mV. Thus chloride ions are very far from equilibrium. The initial conclusion is that there is active transport of chloride inwards at either the plasmalemma or tonoplast or at both. Acceptance of later values of 10 mN for the chloride activity in flowing cytoplasm of Characean plants where the potential distribution is similar (Coster, 1966; Kishimoto and Tazawa, 1965) would mean that chloride is actively transported inwards at both these membranes.

It seems likely that the chloride concentration in the chloroplasts of *Nitella* and *Chara* is higher than in the cytoplasm, probably several hundred mM. Whether this is related to anion exchange properties of the chloroplast or to an active transport system is not known.

(d) Corresponding conclusions for Na^+ and K^+ at the tonoplast can be drawn from the remainder of Table 6.1. Since a 5–6 mV difference between ψ_K and ψ_{obs} (tonoplast) is probably not significant, potassium ions may be passively distributed across the tonoplast. Active transport of Na^+ is required in the direction cytoplasm to vacuole.

6.3 OTHER CELLS

There are several other studies in which reasonable firm conclusions can be drawn from the Nernst criterion. These are summarised in Table 6.2. With higher plants the estimation of ionic and electric

Table 6.2   INDICATIONS OF ACTIVE TRANSPORT FROM CONSIDERATION OF NERNST POTENTIALS AND OBSERVED P.D.S

Cells	Ion	c_o	c_v	ψ_j	ψ_{vo}	Active transport	Reference
Nitellopsis	K	0·65	113	−130		—	MacRobbie
obtusa	Na	30	54	−15	−120 to −200	Out	and Dainty (1958)
	Cl	35	206	+45		In	
Chara	K	0·1	66	−157*	−159	0	Hope and
australis	Na	1·0	53	−93*		Out	Walker (1960)
Chaetomorpha	K	13	541	−94		In	Dodd,
darwinii	Na	500	25	+76	+10	Out	Pitman and
	Cl	523	601	+3·5		0	West (1966)
Griffithsia	K	10	535	−100		In	Findlay,
pulvinata	Na	490	30	+70	−52	Out	Hope and
	Cl	573	606	+1·5		In	Williams (1969)
		a_o	a_{cyt}	ψ_K	ψ_{co}		
Chara	K	0·098	110	−178	−173	0	Vorobiev
australis							(1967)

* Activity ratio γ_v/γ_o taken as 0·76.

gradients are a great deal more difficult and conclusions less clear-cut (see Higinbotham, Etherton and Foster, 1967).

It seems that, very crudely, we can look on the ionic distribution found between the inside and outside of cells as coming about in the following ways.

(a) Synthesis of protein and/or phospholipid cytoplasmic material.

(b) Exchange of H^+ of protoplasm for K^+, Na^+ (outside) across membranes permeable to these ions.

(c) Operation of the ubiquitous 'sodium pump' makes Na^+ the minority of the counterions in the cytoplasm.

(d) In plant cells vacuolation proceeds at a rate determined by active transport of anions inwards.

(e) The relative permeability of the plasmalemma to K^+ and Na^+ determines the proportion of these ions accompanying the transported anions. The proportion may be further modified by active sodium extrusion from cytoplasm to vacuole.

It is the steady state results of these processes (and, no doubt, many others) which the experimenter examines in the mature cells discussed, active fluxes being balanced by approximately equal passive fluxes so that the net fluxes are zero.

6.4 ELECTROGENIC EFFECTS

There are several ways in which operation of active transport systems could modify the trans-membrane potential difference. When this happens, there is said to be an 'electrogenic pump'.

During the passage of a small current J through a membrane, the p.d. across it may be regarded as having two components, thus:

$$\psi = 58 \log_{10} \frac{K_o + \alpha Na_o}{K_i + \alpha Na_i} + J \cdot r_0 \qquad (6.1)$$

where the first term is the diffusion potential already discussed and r_0 is the membrane resistance for small currents (discussed in the next chapter).

If J could be regarded as a net flux due to active transport of, say, Na^+ or Cl^- which we have just 'switched on', it is seen that ψ may become different from ψ_m (Eq. 5.2) owing to one or more of the following effects. (a) Change in K_o or Na_o. (b) Change in K_i or Na_i. (c) Change in α. (d) $J \cdot r_0$, the p.d. due to current through the membrane resistance, may be appreciable. For example, if $r_0 = 10^4 \, \Omega \, cm^2$

and there is a flux $\phi = 10$ pequiv. cm^{-2} s^{-1} ($J \simeq 10^{-6}$ A cm^{-2}), then $J \cdot r_0 = 10$ mV.

Effect (a) may occur in any preparation, in principle, but is particularly likely when the medium is of low concentration and when a cell wall is present. The active transport either depletes or enhances the concentration of the transported ion (and any other ion accompanying it to preserve electric neutrality). This perturbation in the external concentrations would in most situations quickly be made good by diffusion up to, or away from, the membrane. The relative magnitudes of transport and diffusion determine the steady local concentrations just outside the membrane. In so far as the ionic regime within plant cell walls is only slowly changed via changes in the external medium under some conditions (Chapter 5), the effect under discussion will be more important in plant cells and in dilute media.

To take a specific example, initiation of active inward transport of bicarbonate ions, accompanied by K^+, caused the p.d. in *Chara* cells to change from about -160 mV to -200 or more (Hope, 1965). At the time this was attributed to effects (c) and (d) above, but depletion of K^+ just outside the plasmalemma would also have contributed to the observed hyperpolarisation. The relative changes in K_i and Na_i will be much smaller since the cells usually have higher concentrations of these ions in the vacuole and cytoplasm.

Briggs (1962) has worked out one way of finding the effect of extra passive fluxes of ions accompanying an active transport flux. To do this it was necessary to assume a linear potential gradient in the membrane (Chapter 1) so that the net flux of, say, potassium would be

$$\phi_K = -P_K \frac{F\psi_m}{RT} \frac{K_o - K_i \exp(F\psi_m/RT)}{1 - \exp(F\psi_m/RT)} \qquad (6.2)$$

with a similar expression for ϕ_{Na}. Then it was supposed that there was a constant active influx of Cl^- or efflux of Na^+, Φ, such that

$$\Phi = \phi_K + \phi_{Na} \qquad (6.3)$$

Then it could be shown that

$$K_o + \alpha Na_o = (K_i + \alpha Na_i) \exp(F\psi_m/RT)$$
$$- \frac{RT}{F\psi_m} \frac{\Phi}{P_K} [1 - \exp(F\psi_m/RT)] \quad (6.4)$$

To use this equation, reasonable values for $K_i + \alpha Na_i$, α and P_K

have to be assumed and ψ_m has to be solved for (by trial and error) for various Φ. P_K can be estimated from data on flux or on electric resistance of membranes (as outlined in the next chapter) but once again only by following Goldman's arbitrary assumption as to the membrane field. It is sufficient to say here that both Eq. (6.1) and Eq. (6.4) show that active flux as large as 4 pequiv. $cm^{-2} s^{-1}$ (almost the largest chloride influx observed in *Chara*, for example) lead to a more negative potential, 4 mV more negative when $K_o = 0.1$, $Na_o = 1.0$ mN, and only about 1 mV more negative when $K_o = 1.0$, $Na = 0.1$ mN.

Genuine electrogenic effects have been reported in at least two widely different systems, in fungal mycelium (Slayman, 1965) and *Acetabularia* (Saddler, unpublished results). In the latter a light-stimulated chloride flux of several hundred pmol $cm^{-2} s^{-1}$ is associated with a change in the plasmalemma p.d. from somewhere near the potassium equilibrium level of -80 mV in the dark to -160 mV in the light, a spectacular increase.

6.5 THE FLUX RATIO CRITERION

In those situations where the influx and efflux of an ion species are unequal, the Nernst criterion is inappropriate for testing for active transport. Unfortunately, many of the applications of the idea of the equilibrium p.d. have been made in experimental situations where in fact flux measurements of the required accuracy have not been performed in conjunction with those of p.d., ion activity, etc.

Koefoed-Johnsen, Levi and Ussing (1952) made measurements of unidirectional fluxes across frog skin with Ringer's solution on the inside and 1/10 Ringer's on the outside. Isolated frog skin transports NaCl inwards. During the process the inside of the skin is electrically positive to the outside. For chloride ions convincing agreement was obtained between the ratios calculated from the simple flux ratio equation (Chapter 1) and the observations. Table 6.3 presents some of these observations. Adrenalin caused deviations between expected and observed flux ratios, possibly through causing a flux of water. In ion exchange membranes, water fluxes may interact with ion fluxes (cf. Table 3.4). In contrast to the fluxes of chloride, those of sodium were in quite the wrong ratio to be merely the result of the gradient of electrochemical potential. Hence, sodium is actively transported inwards across the frog skin. Numerous sequels to these now classical experiments are to be found in the literature (see Ussing, 1965).

In coenocytes of *Valonia ventricosa* Gutknecht (1966) found that the influx of K^+ and Cl^- exceeded the efflux. The net influx corresponded to a small rate of enlargement of the cells of about 1 % per day. The vacuole concentrations were constant for many days. A potential difference of -71 mV said to refer to the cytoplasm of the coenocytes was in fact measured on aplanospores. Both fluxes and p.d. in Table 6.4 are between sea-water and the vacuole. Table 6.4 shows the results of applying the simple flux ratio relationship to the fluxes of K^+, Na^+ and Cl^- in *Valonia*.

The conclusions for *Valonia* are that (a) there must be inward active transport of K^+ somewhere between the medium and vacuole; (b) there must be outward active transport of Na^+; and (c) chloride ions are passively distributed. In this *Valonia* is similar to *Chaetomorpha* (Table 6.2).

6.6 THE SHORT-CIRCUITING TECHNIQUE

A third method of testing for active transport is to measure the current needed to short-circuit a preparation having similar solution on each side of the transporting membrane or cells. At the same time the fluxes are measured to see which contribute to the short-circuit current. Any net fluxes detected should be due to active transport, because the electrochemical gradients for all ions have been *reduced to zero* ($\Delta\psi = 0$, $c_o = c_i$).

The technique is suitable for preparations where the 'inside' can be perfused with a solution like that outside. Fortunately, some marine coenocytes are large and tolerant enough for this. The short-circuiting procedure was, however, first used with frog skin by Ussing and Zerahn (1951).

Table 6.5 shows a sample of short-circuit currents and fluxes of sodium in an experiment with frog skin. It is apparent that something causes a net flux of sodium from outside to inside in the absence of the more readily understandable forces.

Using giant coenocytes of *Halicystis ovalis*, Blount and Levedahl (1960) were able to perfuse the vacuoles with sea-water under a small pressure, short-circuit the still-persisting p.d., and measure, one at a time, sodium influx and efflux and chloride influx and efflux. Under these conditions there was a net efflux of sodium of approximately 70 pequiv. $cm^{-2} s^{-1}$ when the short-circuit current

Table 6.3 FLUXES (μequiv. cm^{-2} h^{-1}) AND FLUX RATIOS OF CHLORIDE IONS IN FROG SKIN: $Cl_o = 10.6$ mN, $Cl_i = 115$ mN.
(FROM DATA OF KOEFORD-JOHNSEN, LEVI AND USSING, 1952)

ϕ	ϕ_o	$\psi_{io}(mV)$	$(\phi_1/_o)_{obs}$	$(\phi_1/\phi_o)_{calc}$*
0·58	0·15	89	3·85	3·5
0·29	0·069	94	4·2	4·2
0·25	0·065	86	3·9	3·2
0·20	0·052	93	3·9	4·1
0·29	0·052	90	5·7	3·8
0·24	0·047	96	5·2	5·4

* Using activities, not concentrations; $\gamma_o/\gamma_i \simeq 1.1$ for chloride, according to the authors.

Table 6.4 FLUXES AND ION DISTRIBUTION IN *Valonia ventricosa* (GUTKNECHT, 1966)

	c_o	c_v	ϕ_{ov}	ϕ_{vo}	ϕ_{ov}/ϕ_{vo}	ψ_{ov}	$(c_o/c_v)\exp-(zF\psi_{ov}/RT)$
K^+	12	625	88·7	86·2	1·0$_3$	—	0·01
Na^+	508	44	3·6$_4$	3·3$_2$	1·1$_0$	+17	5·8
Cl^-	596	643	18·5	10·9	1·7$_0$	—	1·8

The concentration ratio is approximately the activity ratio since the ionic strengths of vacuole and sea-water are similar.

Table 6.5 SODIUM FLUXES AND SHORT-CIRCUIT CURRENTS IN FROG SKIN
(IN mC cm^{-2} h^{-1}). (FROM DATA OF USSING AND ZERAHN, 1951)

Expt	1		2			3		
Influx	102	93	177	176	124	64	64	57
Current	99	99	174	162	123	63	55	49

Expt	4		5		6	
Efflux	9·7	11·5	5—14		6·0	5·6
Current	130	139	108—112		136	124

was 10–13 μA cm^{-2}. In apparently comparable experiments the short-circuit current was 39–50 μA cm^{-2} and a net influx of chloride of about 200–300 pequiv. cm^{-2} s^{-1} was detected. It was provisionally concluded that net chloride influx and net sodium efflux, when added, nearly accounted for the short-circuit current. Thus sodium and chloride ions are actively transported outwards and inwards, respectively, whereas potassium ions are in electrochemical equilibrium, as far as the incomplete data indicate (cytoplasm activities are not yet available).

Gutknecht (1967) perfused and short-circuited cells of *Valonia ventricosa*, 0·8–1·5 cm in diameter; he found that the short-circuit current was almost twice as large as could be accounted for by the observed net influxes of K$^+$, Cl$^-$ and Na$^+$. A further unresolved difficulty is the very fact that a net chloride influx occurred under these conditions. In normal *Valonia* cells (Gutknecht, 1966) chloride is apparently passively distributed, as we have seen (Table 6.4). Release of hydrostatic pressure or some other factor may cause a large active transport of chloride under the perfused conditions.

6.7 CONCLUSIONS

In this chapter we have concluded that a variety of studies reveal the distribution of ions between the inside and outside of cells to be the result of both passive and active transport. The most common deviation from a passive distribution is found in the level of sodium within cells; this is clearly kept low in comparison with potassium. Although the permeability of most cell membranes to sodium is low compared to potassium and although sodium ions have a surprisingly low activity coefficient in some cells (Chapter 5), this should not prevent an eventual equilibrium in which $a^i_{Na}/a^i_K = a^o_{Na}/a^o_K$. This is not observed and, hence, a special mechanism is invoked named a 'sodium efflux pump' or 'outwardly directed sodium active transport'.

Other ion species are found to be influenced by the metabolism of cells—for example, an influx pump for chloride is common in plant cells.

7

The electric resistance and conductance of cell membranes

7.1 HISTORY

Measurements of the resistance of cells were made more than 30 years ago, in squid axons by Cole and Hodgkin (1939) and in *Valonia* by Blinks (1930), to select two familiar examples. Since then numerous studies of the resistance of cells (attributed, as we shall see, to their membranes) have been made with both direct current and alternating current.

When direct current is injected at a point inside a long cylindrical cell, by being passed through a microelectrode implanted in the cell, the current spreads out in all directions. As shown in Fig. 7.1, the current passes through the surface membrane in decreasing density with increasing distance from the point of injection. This is because the interior of cells has a low but finite resistivity, corresponding approximately to that of a 100–500 mN solution of KCl (c. 89–20Ωcm). The way in which the current density falls off with increasing distance is described by the space constant, or length constant, λ. For a cylinder very long compared with its diameter the current density decays by about 63% for each length constant. In squid giant axons λ is of the order of a millimetre; in *Chara* or *Nitella*, a centimetre. Earlier methods of measuring resistance employed external contacts, not microelectrodes. In these experiments the membrane resistance had to be sorted out from the internal or 'core' resistance by the theory of conduction in insulated cables. It is not surprising that in later experiments long, axial electrodes were employed to ensure that current was passed uniformly through a known area of membrane. A known length of both internal and external solution must be equipotential. Then the change in p.d.

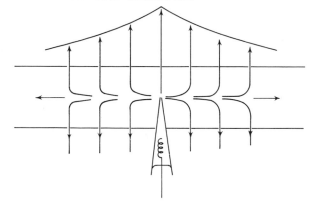

Fig. 7.1   *A diagrammatic representation of the current flow between a point inside a long, cylindrical conductor bounded by an imperfectly insulating surface, and a return circuit consisting of a coil or plate outside lying parallel to the cylinder*

across the membrane measured close to the membrane surfaces in that area is related directly to the resistance.

The methods described lead to a reasonably restricted range of values for the resistance for a unit area of membrane. The range 1000–10 000 $\Omega\,cm^2$ covers a large number of different membranes.

Table 7.1 lists some representative values.

7.2   RELATION BETWEEN CONDUCTANCE AND MEMBRANE PROPERTIES

The measurement of the electric conductance of membranes should yield information about their structure and organisation and about the way ions permeate. However, conductance in an aqueous medium is proportional both to ion mobility and to concentration. Therefore a single measurement of membrane conductance does not enable conclusions to be drawn about the mobility or concentration of ions within the membrane. Nevertheless Cole (1965) was able to estimate the mobility of potassium in the squid axon membranes by an indirect method.

This method depended on measurements of the impedance of axons to alternating current, a subject well reviewed by Cole (Cole, 1962, 1965; Schwan and Cole, 1960). A characteristic frequency was observed to be related to a time for redistribution of the electric field in the membrane. In so far as the main carriers of current are

Table 7.1 THE RESTING RESISTANCE (r_0 in cm^2) OF MEMBRANES IN VARIOUS CELLS MEASURED IN THE MEDIUM INDICATED

Membrane	Medium	r_0	Ref.
Animals			
Squid axon (*Loligo*)	SW	700	Cole and Hodgkin (1939)
Carcinus axon	SW	8000	Hodgkin (1947)
Muscle fibres (*Rana temporaria*)	Ringer's	4000	Hodgkin and Horowicz (1959 a)
Egg cells (*Asterias*)		3100	Tyler et al. (1956)
Resting electroplaques (*Electrophorus electricus*)	SW	7	Whittam and Guinnebault (1959)
Nucleus (*Drosophila flavorepleta*)	—	1	Loewenstein and Kanno (1963)
Plants			
Valonia	SW	5K	Blinks (1930)
Chara	1 mN NaCl / 0·1 mN KCl	15K	Walker (1960)
Chara	1·0 mN NaCl / 0·5 mN CaCl₂	12K(P) / 1K(T)	Findlay and Hope (1964)
Nitella	0·1 mN KCl / 0·1 mN NaCl / 0·2 mN CaCl₂	21K	Williams, Johnston and Dainty (1964)
Griffithsia	SW	200(P) / 5K(T)	Findlay, Hope and Williams (1969)
Avena coleoptiles	1 mN KCl	1300	Higinbotham, Hope and Findlay (1964)
Root hairs (cucumber, etc.)	1 mN KCl + 1 mN CaCl₂	3000(P) / ≃500(T)	Greenham (1966)

K is 'kilo'; SW, sea-water; P, plasmalemma; T, tonoplast.

potassium ions (Chapters 5 and 6). this time constant of 3 ms is related by theory to potassium mobility u_K through

$$\tau_D = kT/u_K e^2 X^2 \qquad (7.1)$$

where τ_D is the time constant for the redistribution of the field, k is Boltzmann's constant, e is the electronic charge and X is the electric field strength. From Eq. (7.1) u_K was found to be 10^{-8} cm^2 s^{-1} V^{-1}. Finally it was argued that a resting membrane resistance of 1000 Ω cm^2 must correspond to that of a thin layer of material (100Å) with K$^+$ at an average concentration of 1 mN and with the stated mobility, which is c. 10^{-5} of that in acqueous solutions. Admittedly approximate, these estimates seem to be the only ones available.

7.3 THE RELATION BETWEEN CONDUCTANCE AND ION FLUXES

7.3.1 Large currents

When an electric current is passed through a cell membrane, the current must correspond to the movement of charges on one or more of the following:

cations: K$^+$, Na$^+$, Ca^{++}, Mg^{++}, H$^+$, etc.

anions: Cl$^-$, SO$_4^=$, Br$^-$, NO$_3^-$, etc.

electrons

In certain situations it has clearly been shown that specified ions carry most of an applied current; for example, potassium ions carry outward current in squid giant axons. Figure 7.2 illustrates this. In the experiments the axon membrane was subjected to estimated depolarisations of up to 50 mV.

7.3.2 Resting flux and the conductance with small currents

At a membrane potential at which a particular ion species is at electrochemical equilibrium it was shown that a flux ϕ_j (influx or efflux) contributes a partial ion conductance, *when there is independent ion migration* (defined in Chapter 1):

$$g_j = (Z_j^2 F^2/RT)\phi_j \qquad (7.2)$$

Such a relation fails dismally to account for any but a fraction of the plasmalemma conductance in Characean cells, where, for example, $\phi_K \sim 1$ pequiv. cm^{-2} s^{-1} and g_K from Eq. (7.2) = 4 μmho cm^{-2} of a total conductance of 50–100 μmho cm^{-2} (Table 7.1). The fluxes of Na$^+$, Cl$^-$ and Ca^{++} would not yield more than an additional few μmho, but there is no justification for using Eq. (7.2) for ions not near

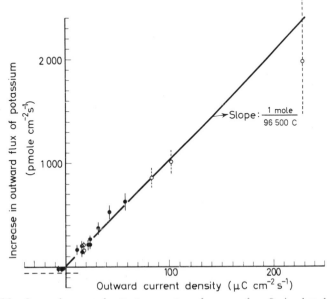

Fig. 7.2   *Outward current density in a portion of an axon from* Sepia *plotted against increase in efflux of potassium ions* (Fig. 4, *Hodgkin and Huxley, 1953*). *The standard errors shown were mainly due to counting errors in the estimation of radioactivity. The open circles were got by a method of estimation different from that used for the other points. The resting efflux or 'leakage' was* 55 pequiv. cm^{-2} s^{-1}, *which level is shown as a dotted line.* (*Reproduced by kind permission of the authors and of* The Journal of Physiology)

equilibrium. Nor is the situation happier when squid axons are considered: for $K_o = 10.4$ mM, $\phi_K \simeq 5$ at $\psi_m = \psi_K(-74$ mV$)$ in certain experiments made by Hodgkin and Keynes (1955). Thus g_K (Eq. 7.2) = 0.02 mmho cm^{-2} when the membrane electrical conductance would have been about 0.5 mmho cm^{-2}. For an axon depolarised with 104 mN K$^+$ outside, the influx and efflux were 170 pequiv. cm^{-2} s^{-1}, g_K (Eq. 7.2) was 0.66, but the electric conductance was 3 mmho cm^{-2}. (These axons were treated with DNP to abolish a component of potassium influx coupled with active sodium extrusion.)

An artibrary constant n' was introduced in the discussion of these results, which when used in Eq. (7.1) predicted roughly the correct conductance under some conditions (although apparently not for the resting flux when K_o was 10·4 mN), i.e.

$$g_K = n'(F^2/RT)\phi_K \qquad (7.3)$$

n' was 2–4 in *Sepia* axons. It was clear from this and other considerations of flux as a function of p.d. that the movements of potassium ions in axon membranes were not 'independent'. There will be occasion to return to those experiments in the next chapter, on ionic fluxes.

Further indications that potassium ions are the main current-carriers in the plasmalemma in *Chara* and *Griffithsia* cells resulted

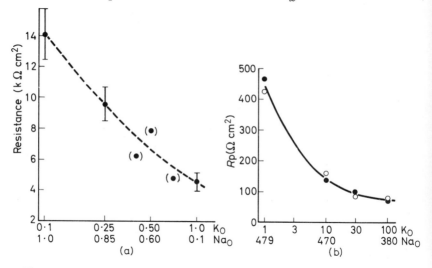

Fig. 7.3   (a) *The electric resistance between the vacuole and external medium of* Chara *cells, in media in which* K_o *and* Na_o *are varied but* $K_o + Na_o$ *kept constant at* 1·1 mN. *The bracketed points are means of only 2–3 values; the other points are means with S.E.M. of 5 values.* (Replotted from data of Hope and Walker, 1961. *Reproduced by kind permission of* Australian Journal of Biological Sciences) (b) *The resistance of the plasmalemma of two* Griffithsia *cells in artificial sea-waters containing the potassium and sodium levels indicated.* (Data from Findlay, Hope and Williams, 1969)

from measurements of resistance as a function of external concentration of potassium and sodium. Figure 7.3 shows that added potassium decreased the resistance. Presumably the ionic regime within the plasmalemma was changed to include more of the most mobile species, namely potassium.

7.4 CONDUCTANCE OF 'INTERNAL' MEMBRANES

The enveloping membrane of mitochondria plainly has a high but unmeasurable resistance compared with the interior, as is shown by the electrical behaviour of suspensions of mitochondria in an alternating current field (Hope, 1956; Pauly, Packer and Schwan, 1960). The capacitance per unit area is similar to that of some other surface membranes.

The resistance of the membranes of nuclei has been measured directly (e.g. by Loewenstein and Kanno, 1963) with inserted microelectrodes. The nuclei of gland cells of several insect genera have membranes with an area specific resistance of close to $1\ \Omega\ cm^2$. Considering the large pores visible in electron micrographs of the nuclear membrane in numerous cells, the resistance is surprisingly high. The membrane separates cytoplasm and nucleoplasm, each assumed to have a resistivity of about $100\ \Omega$ cm. It is concluded that the pores in the nuclear membrane are not filled with material of this resistivity, otherwise the trans-membrane resistance should be $1\ m\Omega\ cm^2$. This is a notable discrepancy between results from studies of structure and function.

Although the surface membrane of epithelial cells has a high resistance ($10^4\ \Omega\ cm^2$), Locwenstein and Kanno (1964) found that current passed relatively freely through the junction of two adjoining cells from *Drosphila* salivary gland. Many dyes as well as ions were able to diffuse between cells. The ease of 'communication' between cells is apparently connected with a low level of intracellular Ca^{++}. Significantly, cancer cells were found to have a much reduced conductance at adjoining boundaries between cells, and a higher than normal external surface resistance (Loewenstein and Kanno, 1966).

7.5 RECTIFICATION

When current is passed through the membranes of *Chara* cells, most of the change in p.d. occurs at the plasmalemma, because the resistance of the tonoplast is much lower (Table 7.1). Thus data on the resistance or p.d. vs. current density obtained in this way relate fairly well to the plasmalemma. Figure 7.4 reproduces data of this sort. There was little theoretical background when these experiments were done (time has not improved matters) and the authors used the Goldman assumption to calculate a relationship between resistance and membrane potential for the simple model where there is voltage-invariant permeability to K^+ and Na^+ only. If the measured resistance r were $\Delta\psi/J$ it could be shown that

$$r = \frac{RT\Delta\psi[1 - \exp(F\psi/RT)]}{F^2\psi(P_K K_o + P_{Na} Na_o)[1 - \exp(F\Delta\psi/RT)]} \qquad (7.4)$$

where $\Delta\psi$ is the change in membrane p.d. from the resting value and ψ the p.d. reached on applying the current. Equation (7.4) corresponds to Eq. 1.20. The full line in Fig. 7.4 shows that Eq. (7.4) describes the variation in r reasonably well if $P_K \simeq 10^{-5}$ cm s^{-1} and $\alpha \simeq 0.1$.

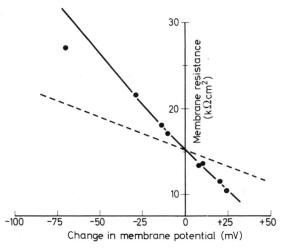

Fig. 7.4   *The resistance of* Chara *cell membranes (plasmalemma and tonoplast in series) as a function of the change in p.d. caused by an applied current. The full line was calculated according to Eq. (7.4), the dotted line from another theory. (From Hope and Walker, 1961. Reproduced by kind permission of* Australian Journal of Biological Sciences)

Another relation between r and ψ based on Planck's assumption (of microscopic electroneutrality everywhere in the membrane) is less successful, as the dotted line reveals.

Coster (1965) extended this study to a wider range of ψ, mainly in the hyperpolarising direction since action potentials may intervene during substantial depolarisations. Figure 7.5 gives an example of the relation between ψ and J (a) for both cytoplasmic membranes in series, and (b) for the plasmalemma alone. The membrane p.d. cannot be polarised past about 300 mV, even with very large currents. This phenomenon was termed 'punch-through', by analogy with a well-known effect in semiconductor devices. It has been

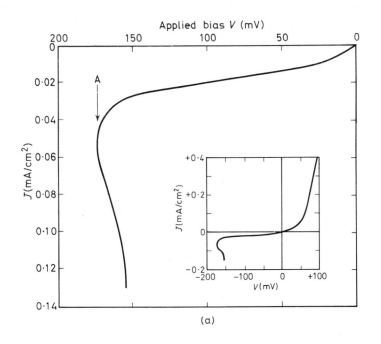

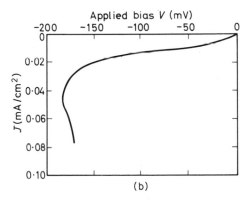

Fig. 7.5 (a) *The variation of membrane potential difference with current in a cell of* Chara australis, *recording from the vacuole. The* change *in potential is V. The resting potential was* −125 mV. '*Punch through' occurred at A when the p.d. was* −300 mV. *The inset shows the depolarising direction of p.d. change as well.* (b) *The p.d. vs. current relationship for the plasmalemma alone (recording from the cytoplasm) in a* Chara *cell.* (*From Coster, 1965. Reproduced by kind permission of the author and of the Rockefeller Institute Press, publishers of* Biophysical Journal)

observed in several genera of plants. Such a discontinuity in the J vs. ψ curve is certainly not predicted by the simple Goldman-based model but is expected if the cell membrane is composed of apposed layers of opposite fixed charge. Between these layers, if they are close enough, there is a 'depletion layer' in which each type of counter-ion is repelled into the fixed-charge region by the field of the fixed charges in the opposite side (Fig. 7.6). When an appropriate bias is

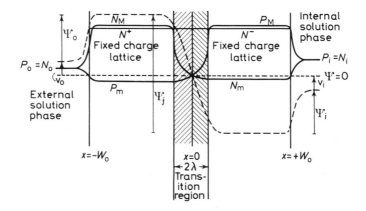

Fig. 7.6 *Double-lattice, fixed-charge membrane in which the region between $x = -W_o$ and $x = 0$ has fixed positive charges and is in contact with the region between $x = 0$ and $x = +W_o$ which contains fixed negative charges. The profiles for the mobile ion concentrations and the electrostatic potential, ψ, are shown qualitatively. $\psi = 0$ is taken arbitrarily at $x = 0$ as shown. Note that the trans-membrane potential equals $V_o + V_i$. The profiles for the concentration of mobile ions do not necessarily cross exactly at the point $\psi = 0$. (From Coster, 1965. Reproduced by kind permission of the author and of the Rockefeller University Press, publishers of the* Biophysical Journal)

applied to such a compound membrane, the depletion layer increases in width until it extends to the outer edges of the membrane. There is then a sudden increase in current. There is rather satisfactory agreement between the punch-through potential observed and that predicted from the theory of the double, fixed-charge membrane, if several plausible assumptions are made about charge density and dielectric constant in the membrane. In addition rectification of about the observed amount also results from the theory. It was found from experiments with radioactive tracers that a large efflux of chloride ions accounted for the current in the region of punch-through. The chloride conductance will be referred to again in a later chapter.

7.6 ELECTROKINETIC PHENOMENA

7.6.1 Introduction

There have been few studies of electro-osmosis and streaming potentials in cells or in biological membranes. This is probably because the water flows that accompany the moderate electric currents tolerated by cell membranes are small and difficult to measure.

We saw in Chapters 2 and 3 that frictional interactions between ions and water may lead to (a) a streaming current or potential when water flow is caused by a gradient of osmotic potential or hydrostatic pressure or (b) a water flow when a stream of ions is caused to pass through a membrane by an electric field. Thus the very appearance of an electro-osmotic water flow might be taken to be evidence for ion migration through a membrane in regions where a water flux was also possible.

7.6.2 Electro-osmosis in Characean cells

Fensom and Dainty (1963) reported electro-osmotic water flows in *Nitella* cells amounting to about 20 µl H_2O per coulomb or approximately 100 mol H_2O per faraday. This last figure is identical with 100 molecules of H_2O per monovalent ion, an enormous interaction. The water flow occurred in the direction of positive ion current.

The phenomenon, but not the interpretation, was confirmed by Barry (1967) after a careful study of *Chara* cells. The complex nature of the system through which current is passed prompts a thorough examination of the possible causes of a current-induced water flow. There are two surface membranes, the cytoplasm and the cell wall, to be considered. Briggs (1967) has pointed out that electro-osmosis in the cell wall alone might be sufficient to cause a volume flow through an adhering lipid membrane when the latter was water-permeable but ions and water followed separate paths in it. Barry and Hope (1969 a) have pointed out that local osmosis occurs across a membrane when there is a discontinuity at the membrane surface in the transport number of the ion carrying most of the membrane current. The perturbations in the concentration caused by this discontinuity have been referred to as a probable factor in so-called electrogenic pumps (Chapter 6). The effect may also lead to underestimation of ion fluxes (Chapter 8). These effects will now be briefly discussed.

7.6.3 The cell wall

Table 7.2 lists some of the relevant properties of isolated cell walls and the same parameters for intact cells. As is to be expected of a structure containing charged, narrow interstices filled with electrolyte, the cell wall shows electro-osmosis. Will a composite 'membrane' composed of cell wall and adhering lipo-protein membrane

Table 7.2 OSMOTIC AND ELECTRO-OSMOTIC CHARACTERISTICS OF CELLS OF *Nitella* AND *Chara*

	Walls	Intact cells	Ref.
Hydraulic conductivity (L_p) (cm s^{-1} atm^{-1})	$1.8-3.5 \times 10^{-5}$	—	Tazawa and Kamiya (1966)
	$3.1-4.0 \times 10^{-5}$	—	Barry and Hope (1969 b)
		1.0×10^{-5}	Dainty and Ginzburg (1964)
		1.0×10^{-5}	Barry and Hope (1969 b)
Electro-osmotic permeability $(\beta,$ cm^3 C$^{-1})$	0.011	0.0076	Barry and Hope (1969 b)
Maximum volume flow due to local osmosis $(\alpha,$ cm^3 C$^{-1})$	0.023	$0.01-0.02$	Barry and Hope (1969 b)
Total current-induced volume flow $(\alpha + \beta)$	—	0.019	Fensom and Dainty (1963)
	—	0.017	Barry and Hope (1969 b)

show this property as well, if only the cell wall has coupling between ion and water movement? The answer is 'yes', because electro-osmotic water flow causes a pressure gradient across the cell wall unless the cell membrane has infinitely high hydraulic conductivity, which is not the case. This is illustrated in the composite membrane model (Fig. 7.7).

7.6.4 Local osmosis

Figure 7.8 shows the changes of concentration expected on each side of a membrane when current through it is carried by, say, K$^+$ with $t_K = 1.0$, while on each side $t_K = t_{Cl} = 0.5$.

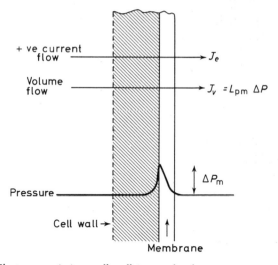

Fig. 7.7 *Electro-osmosis in a cell wall is postulated to cause a pressure difference across an adhering lipo-protein membrane and, hence, water flow through the whole system is caused by a current*

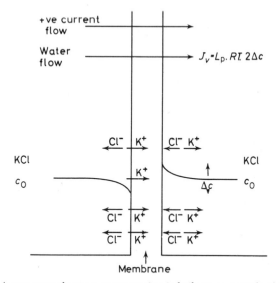

Fig. 7.8 *Across a membrane a concentration is built up as a result of current being carried entirely by potassium ions within the membrane, but distributed between potassium and chloride ions, on each side. The concentration gradient causes local osmosis of the magnitude shown*

The local concentration changes will tend to be dissipated by diffusion and by the osmosis itself. When the current is turned on, the rate of volume flow will increase to a steady level even though true electro-osmosis may be absent. Proper electro-osmosis should appear instantaneously.

Current-induced local osmosis should be of general occurrence but does not seem to have been widely considered. Local osmosis due to concentration gradients being built up by active transport is of importance in the gall-bladder (Diamond and Tormey, 1966) and in secretion by salt glands in mangrove trees (Atkinson *et al.*, 1967).

The current-induced volume flow in *Chara* cells and cell walls can be divided into two components—an instantaneous flow and a steady maximum rate that has developed in the ensuing few minutes (Table 7.2). The rates of 'true' electro-osmosis in walls or in cells are comparable and are 7–10 μl C^{-1}. Calculations for the model of Fig. 7.7 show that the apparent electro-osmotic flow in intact cells (supposing coupling to take place only in cell walls) should be rather less than that observed (2·9 μl C^{-1} calculated, 7μl C^{-1} observed). Nevertheless the existence of water-filled pores through which ions migrate is not proven beyond doubt by these experiments.

7.6.5   Streaming potentials

Diamond (1962) and Pidot and Diamond (1964) reported that potential differences were observed across gall-bladder preparations when sucrose + Ringer's solution on one side caused a water flow from Ringer's solution on the other side. The streaming potential built up with a half-time of about 7 s (Diamond 1966) following the addition of sucrose.

In this instance a possible extra diffusion potential due to enhancement and depletion of concentrations was shown to be absent. This was proved as follows: a p.d. change was observed when 200 mN NaCl on each side was modified to 200 mN (serosal) and 50 mN NaCl + 300 m OsM sucrose (mucosal). The mucosal side became 7 mV positive when the change was made, with zero water flow, or with a large water flow caused by an osmotic gradient. A genuine streaming potential such as that observed in the gall-bladder preparation is evidence of water flow through channels containing a negative fixed charge.

7.7   CONCLUSIONS

The types of experiment which have been outlined in this chapter allow several fairly general conclusions to be made about cells and membranes. These are as follows.

(a) There is a resistance to the flow of electricity at the boundary of cell protoplasm, both with the environment (animal and plant cells) and with the vacuole (plants). This is highly significant in relation to theories that seek to explain ionic relations in terms of adsorption-exchange and restricted diffusion within cytoplasm.

(b) The resting conductance of a unit area of surface membranes of cells of many sorts is $0.1-1$ mmho cm^{-2}. The lower conductance of some plant cell membranes is almost certainly associated with the fact that the normal ionic environment is much more dilute than sea-water, blood plasma, etc. Marine coenocytes are more like animal cells in respect of their membrane conductance. A conductance of the order of 1 mmho cm^{-2} corresponds to a resistivity of 10^9 Ω cm in a structure 100Å thick. This is large compared with the resistivity of the environment (20–1000 Ω cm), the vacuole (100 Ω cm) or the bulk of the protoplasm (100 Ω cm). On the last-named there is only indirect evidence (see Chapter 6).

(c) Ions such as K$^+$, Na$^+$ and Cl$^-$ and not electrons or protons conduct electric charge through surface membranes. This is not to say that cell membranes are impermeable to protons, but their concentration usually is small compared with that of the other ions.

(d) The conductance of membranes can be altered by altering the concentration of ions outside the cells or by altering the potential difference across the membrane. This suggests changes in the ion regime inside the membrane or at 'gates' on the surfaces, and subtle changes in membrane structure.

(e) Preferential permeability to K$^+$ and Na$^+$ (compared with Cl$^-$) in some cells in their 'resting state' suggests that part of the membrane may have cation exchange properties (negative indiffusible charges). The phenomenon of 'punch-through' and the vastly increased chloride conductance in some membranes, when they are hyperpolarised, suggests regions of positive and negative fixed charge arranged in sandwich fashion.

Still other cells are preferentially permeable to chloride ions. In muscle fibres the chloride permeability may be associated with a transverse tubular system that has communication with the extracellular fluid parallel with the surface membrane (Girardier et al., 1963). The resting potassium permeation is associated with the surface membrane.

8

Ion fluxes

8.1 INTRODUCTION

Reference has already been made to fluxes of ions under various headings. In this chapter an attempt is made to give a picture of the traffic of ions in and out of cells as revealed by measurements of fluxes. In Chapter 1 the methods used to estimate unidirectional fluxes were outlined. If the fluxes to be measured were in and out of a single compartment, both sides of which were accessible, the job would be comparatively easy. As it is, real cells of experimental fame have Schwann cells (axons), nodal cells (*Nitella*) and cell walls (plants), which complicate the interpretation of data. In addition plant cells have two internal macro-compartments, cytoplasm and vacuole, and all cells have other compartments, micro-compartments, such as chloroplasts and/or mitochondria which possibly cause further departures from the model assumed. Hence, the procedures from which the conclusions of the present chapter have been distilled are devious or complicated. The conclusions are correspondingly a first approximation and it is not surprising that some aspects are still controversial.

8.2 RESTING FLUXES IN GIANT AXONS

When isolated axons are put in sea-water containing radioactive K^+ or Na^+ and subsequently counted whole with a radiation detector, the count does not give a measure of the flux into the axon proper because of substantial amounts of radioactivity located in an extra-axonal compartment, probably in Schwann cells. Other extracellular, diffusible radioactivity will be washed away by brief rinsing with sea-water. More reliable estimates of influx have come from determinations of radioactivity in the isolated axoplasm after the rinsing period. The unidirectional fluxes found in *Sepia* and *Loligo* are shown in Fig. 8.1.

The size of the potassium flux in squid axons and the amount of K^+ in the axoplasm are such that the exchange of labelled for unlabelled K^+ has a half-time of about 35 h (a rate constant of c. $0.02\,h^{-1}$ or c. $5 \times 10^{-6}\,s^{-1}$).

It has already been pointed out that a substantial part of the sodium efflux in many cells must be active and the same is true of

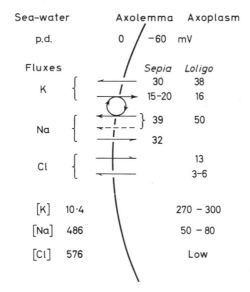

Fig. 8.1 *Mean concentrations and fluxes in giant axons from* Sepia *and* Loligo. *The concentrations are* mequiv. l^{-1}, *and fluxes in* pequiv. $cm^{-2}\,s^{-1}$. (*Data of Hodgkin and Keynes, 1955 a*)

giant axons. Similarly, some of the potassium influx is taken to be active and indeed coupled in some way to the sodium efflux. Evidence for this comes from the effect of removal of external K^+, which lowers $Na\phi_o$ by 2/3 (*Sepia*). Low temperature also reduces $Na\phi_o$ and $K\phi_i$ by similar amounts; the temperature effect on these fluxes has a high $Q_{10}(3-4)$, suggestive of a mediation by metabolic reactions. By contrast, the Q_{10} for $Na\phi_i$ and $K\phi_o$ is lower (1.1–1.4). These fluxes are passive fluxes in the direction of the gradients of electrochemical potential.

The effects on fluxes of inhibitors of metabolism such as 2,4-dinitrophenol, sodium azide, etc., are relegated to a later chapter.

During excitation, as is well known, extra fluxes of K^+ and Na^+ occur in the 'downhill' directions. The effect of the active transport is to tend to maintain the electrochemical gradients that 'drive' the fluxes during depolarisation and the conducted spike. Without the active maintenance of these gradients a giant axon could conduct about 500000 impulses, according to Hodgkin (1964), but a small fibre a lot fewer. Saltatory conduction, in which fluxes occur only at the nodes of Ranvier, is an economical use of the K^+/Na^+ battery.

Further data have been obtained from perfused and dialysed axons, in which the passive fluxes ($Na\phi_i$ and $K\phi_o$) are higher but in which the active fluxes are still present, provided that a 'fuel' such as ATP is provided to the inside of the axons. Brinley and Mullins (1967) describe some significant experiments in this area and list a number of other authors' results.

8.3 MUSCLE FIBRES

Single muscle fibres dissected from *Rana temporaria* and used for electrical measurements by Hodgkin and Horowicz (1959 a) were also used by them in an investigation into the movements of sodium and potassium ions (1959 b). The limitations of using whole muscle for studying ion fluxes are apparent—heterogeneity of membrane permeability and diameter, complications of intercellular diffusion, and adsorption of ions in connective tissue. As opposed to this, single fibres are difficult to prepare and may have been subject to damage. In the experiments referred to the fibres were still excitable, and net efflux of K^+ and influx of Na^+ were small in the resting condition, which argues against a damaged state. In single fibres in Ringer's solution there was an influx and efflux of K^+ of 3–6 pequiv. $cm^{-2} s^{-1}$; the unidirectional fluxes of Na^+ were about four of these units. Higher effluxes of K^+ and influxes of Na^+ were, however, observed in fibres a longer time after isolation.

For both sodium and potassium ions the exchange of radioactive for stable isotope corresponded to single-compartment kinetics. That is, the radioactivity of the fibres decreased negative-exponentially with time. This suggested that the exchange was rate-limited by a surface membrane.

Subsequently, Sjodin and Henderson (1964), using whole muscle prepared from the sartorius muscle of *Rana pipiens*, found that the potassium ion exchange was described by a single exponential function. Notwithstanding the well-known complexity of the internal structure of muscle, the surface membrane apparently controls overall ion exchange (of K^+) and any compartmentalisation of the interior is not revealed by this type of experiment.

Ling (see, for example, 1966) has roundly disagreed with the idea that a surface membrane controls Na^+ exchange but agrees that

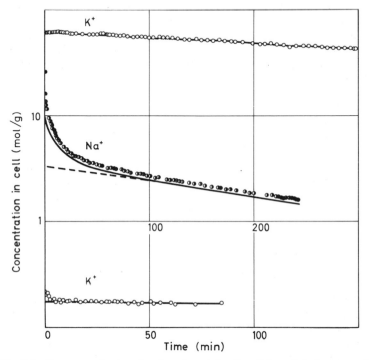

Fig. 8.2 *Frog sartorius muscle: the release of radioactivity, plotted as amount remaining, in chemical units, on a log scale against time. Top curve: the release of potassium from tissue previously loaded for 40 h at 4°C in K^+ - labelled Ringer's solution; efflux at 25°C. Middle curve: sodium efflux at 0°C from tissue loaded for 24 h at 2°C in Na^+ - labelled Ringer's. Bottom curve: potassium efflux at 0°C; tissue loaded at 0°C for 7·9 min. in K^+ - labelled Ringer's. All elutions into phosphate Ringer's. Radioactivity calculated to have originated in extracellular spaces and connective tissue has been allowed for in plotting the full lines. (From Ling, 1966. Reproduced by kind permission of the author and of the New York Academy of Sciences)*

the kinetics of K^+ movement are consistent with membrane control. Sodium ions are claimed to be constrained in their diffusion *within* cytoplasm but not at the surface of cells. Figure 8.2 shows curves of changes in labelled sodium and potassium as functions of time, obtained in frog sartorius muscle. Extracellular sodium is said to have been allowed for. Many other curves similar to the one for sodium have been obtained for the exchange of other ions and of non-electrolytes from labelled muscle.

It may well be that a reduced diffusion coefficient is appropriate for Na^+ in view of Ling's reasoning and in view of the unexpectedly low activity coefficient for sodium in cytoplasm (Lev, 1964—referred to in an earlier chapter). Whether Ling's concept of an ordered, lattice-like fixed-charge system for cytoplasm, with many adjacent layers of ordered water, will turn out to be valid, only time and experiments will tell. In the meantime, Ling's theory is to be found in his book *A physical theory of the living state*.

8.4 PLANT CELLS

Mature cells of plants have two macro-compartments, vacuole and cytoplasm, and two membranes, the tonoplast and the plasmalemma, which might be expected to influence the rate of passage of ions. Both these membranes have been shown to have a low electric conductance relative to the phases they separate, with the proviso that the conductance of the bulk of the cytoplasm is in doubt but can be estimated indirectly.

In principle, as discussed in Chapter 1, a detailed analysis of the curve for the release of radioactive ions from previously labelled plant cells can enable estimation of four quantities, if the cells are in a state of flux equality with no net flux inwards or outwards. These quantities are ϕ_p, ϕ_t, Q_1 and Q_2, where ϕ_p and ϕ_t are the uni-directional fluxes across the plasmalemma and tonoplast, respectively, and Q_1, Q_2 are the quantities of ions in the cytoplasm and vacuole, respectively.

The expected relation is indeed sometimes observed between radioactivity remaining in a cell and time, as seen in Fig. 8.3. In other studies, especially with potassium ions, the log plot remains curved after long times (MacRobbie, 1962: *Nitella translucens*; Dodd, Pitman and West, 1966: *Chaetomorpha darwinii*). When this happens it could be concluded that the long-term rate constant k_L is decreasing for some reason, or that the model is inadequate. Hence, more confidence might be placed in conclusions drawn from direct measurements of cytoplasm and vacuole (Chapter 1, Sub-section 1.8.3).

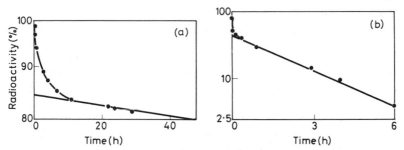

Fig. 8.3 (a) *The release of radioactivity from a cell of* Nitellopsis obtusa *previously soaked in* K^+ *- labelled, brackish water* (K_o = 2–4 mN) *and eluted with the normal medium containing* 0.65 mN K^+. *The activity is on a log scale. The linear portion has been identified as representing exchange of vacuolar potassium.* (b) *When the points for the whole cell in the times 0–6 h are replotted after subtraction of the amounts in the vacuole at those times (obtained from the extrapolate of the linear portion in* (a), *the result is an exponential release (half time,* 1.5–2 h) *preceded by a very rapid release, probably from the cell wall and adhering solution. The linear portion of this graph has been interpreted as exchange of cytoplasmic potassium.* (From *MacRobbie and Dainty,* 1958. *Reproduced by kind permission of the authors and of the Rockefeller Institute Press, publishers of* The Journal of General Physiology)

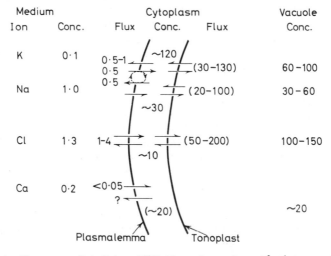

Fig. 8.4 *Characean cells in light at* 18°C. *Fluxes in* pequiv. $cm^{-2} s^{-1}$. *Average figures were taken from MacRobbie* (1962, 1964, 1966 b), *Hope* (1963), *Spanswick and Williams* (1965) *and Coster and Hope* (1968). *The figures in parentheses are in doubt because it is not certain whether ions reaching the vacuole mix with the cytoplasmic ions (see also Sub-section* 8.4.2). *The cytoplasm concentrations refer to the streaming phase. Barr* (1965) *found the* K^+ *and* Na^+ *fluxes (probably* ϕ_p) *in* Nitella clavata *to be lower than those in the figure by a factor of* 10. *This may have been due to a species difference or to the presence of divalent cations in the medium at a concentration of* 2 mM

8.4.1   Fresh-water algae

In some Characean cells measurements of Q_1 have been obtained by chemical analysis of cytoplasm remaining after the vacuole has been perfused away (Kishimoto and Tazawa, 1965). MacRobbie (1962, 1964) has developed methods for determining radioactivity and chemical content of cytoplasm or chloroplasts. By making a synthesis of many such studies, it is possible to give a picture (Fig. 8.4) of the steady state conditions in an 'average cell' of *Nitella* or *Chara*. Metabolic factors that have been found to influence fluxes and membrane properties will be referred to later.

8.4.2   Marine algae

There have been a number of incomplete studies with marine algae. Some results from these have been mentioned already.

Figure 8.5 summarises some of the results obtained with three genera that differ in interesting ways in their ionic relations. In *Griffithsia* spp. the vacuole stores potassium but much less sodium, and the p.d. there is markedly negative. In *Chaetomorpha* and *Valoniopsis* the vacuole is almost equipotential with the medium and chloride ions are nearly in equilibrium (cf. *Valonia*, Table 6.4), but in *Valoniopsis* potassium is not accumulated by more than a factor of 5 and the sodium content is high.

The fluxes into and out of the vacuole are shown in parentheses because there is some doubt as to whether some of the ion flux may not pass through the cytoplasm without exchanging with the cytoplasmic pool of ions. The dotted lines indicate this possible pathway, suggested by MacRobbie (1969) and others to be a vesicular movement, originating at or near the plasmalemma.

In all these algae quite a large flux of potassium occurs at the plasmalemma, corresponding to passive permeation. The sodium flux is low except in *Valoniopsis*, where in addition it is much more variable among cells and collections of cells. Another factor leading to the high vacuolar ratio of $Na^+ : K^+$ is the low flux of potassium into the vacuole, compared with the other genera examined.

Gutknecht and Dainty (1968) give a valuable review of the ionic relations of marine algae.

8.5 THE NON-INDEPENDENCE OF POTASSIUM FLUXES

8.5.1   *Sepia* axons

In Chapter 7 we noted that Hodgkin and Keynes (1955 b) found that the partial conductance due to K^+ was smaller than the observed

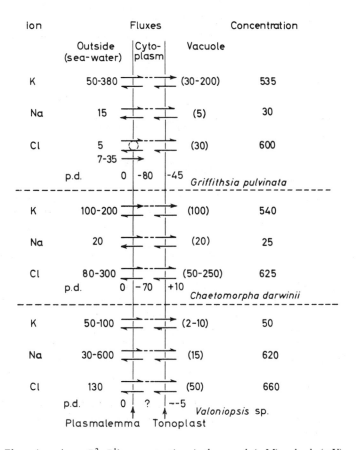

Fig. 8.5 *Fluxes* (pequiv. cm^{-2} s^{-1}), *concentrations in the vacuole* (mM) *and p.d.s* (mV) *in three genera of marine algae. As in Fig. 8.4, and as mentioned in the text, the tonoplast fluxes (in parentheses) are probably minimal. They were calculated by dividing the rate of arrival of vacuolar radioactivity by the external specific activity. This will under-estimate the fluxes across the tonoplast if any mixing with cytoplasmic ions occurs. Data from Dodd, Pitman and West (1966) for* Chaetomorpha (Na$^+$ *and* K$^+$)*, and unpublished data from collaborators acknowledged in the Preface*

electric conductance in axons. Since these ions were strongly indicated as the main current-carriers, this finding clearly pointed to absence of independence in the unidirectional fluxes of potassium. Hodgkin and Keynes made further tests for independence by measuring fluxes when the membrane potential was shifted from the resting level by application of a current. Their aim was to test the now familiar flux ratio equation, which assumes only passive and independent ion migration, i.e.

$$\phi_i/\phi_o = (K_o/K_i) \exp(-F\psi_m/RT) \qquad (8.1)$$

With the Nernst equilibrium potential in mind, we see that Eq. (8.1) transposes readily to

$$\log_{10}(\phi_i/\phi_o) = \frac{\psi_K - \psi_m}{58} \qquad (8.2)$$

(if the ψ are in mV at $T \simeq 18°C$). It is therefore expected that (a) the log of the flux ratio will be a linear function of potential, (b) the flux ratio should change by a factor of 10 for every change of 58 mV in p.d., and (c) the flux ratio should be unity at $\psi_m = \psi_K$. Figure 8.6 (a) shows that in *Sepia* axons the unidirectional fluxes changed in the expected direction when ψ_m was changed, and that their ratio was 1 when $\psi_m = -74$ mV, which is not far from ψ_K.

The log of ϕ_i/ϕ_o was approximately linear with ψ_m, but its slope was some 2–3 times that predicted by Eq. (8.2) (Fig. 8.6b). Beyond all doubt, influx and efflux were not independent. This constant change in the slope of the flux ratio from the 'independent slope' is about equal to the constant factor needed to match the electric conductance with the potassium conductance (Sub-section 7.3, Eq. 7.3).

An empirical measure of the partial conductance can be obtained from data such as those in Fig. 8.6 (a) for any ion since, as seen in Chapter 1,

$$g_j = F(\partial\phi_j/\partial\psi_m) \qquad (8.3)$$

For small changes in p.d. a good approximation would be

$$g'_j = F \,\Delta\phi_j/\Delta\psi_m \qquad (8.4)$$

where ϕ_j is the net flux of ions j.

It is clear that interaction between K^+ fluxes occurs. Hodgkin and Keynes (1955 b) proposed a model in which ions are confined to narrow pores in the membrane, such that a net flux in one direction or other causes a marked reduction of the tracer-measured

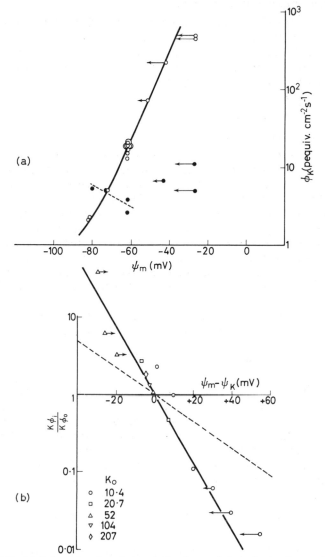

Fig. 8.6   (a) *Influx (closed circles) and efflux (open circles) of potassium, as functions of the membrane p.d. in* Sepia *axons. The arrows show approximate corrections to the estimate for p.d., necessary because of cable effects. Data, replotted, from Hodgkin and Keynes (1955 b). (b) Flux ratios from experiments such as in Fig. 8.6(a), plotted against membrane p.d. The theoretical relationships represented by the lines are discussed in the text. (Data, replotted, from Hodgkin and Keynes, 1955 b. Reproduced by kind permission of the authors and of* The Journal of Physiology)

flux in the opposite direction, compared with independent migration. When the p.d. is changed, however, there is also the possibility of change in fluxes of other ions and of water (through electro-osmosis). These in turn might influence the flux under study, if the interacting fluxes have a pathway in common.

8.5.2   *Chara* and *Nitella*

Influx and efflux of potassium were found to vary with p.d. in *Nitella translucens* and *Chara australis*. In these cells the tonoplast flux is usually high in comparison with that across the plasmalemma (Fig. 8.4). Hence, counts of the whole cell (less cell wall) activity for suitable times serve to estimate ϕ_p. However, vacuolar measurements of p.d. were made and injections of current to change the plasmalemma p.d. were made with a second vacuolar electrode. Because of the relative resistances of the two cytoplasmic surfaces, the change in p.d. across the plasmalemma is about 0·9 of the change measured with an electrode in the vacuole. The length constant was large enough to introduce little error because of cable effects (Chapter 7).

In *Nitella translucens* cells Walker and Hope (1969) showed that the flux ratio varied with p.d. according to the equation

$$\log_{10}(\phi_i/\phi_o) = 2\cdot5\left(\frac{146 - \psi_m}{58}\right)$$

where, again, the log of the flux ratio had a slope 2·5 times that required for independent fluxes. The agreement with the findings for *Sepia* axons is likely to be fortuitous, because there is every reason to believe that influx and efflux were underestimated (see below).

When the partial conductances were calculated for *Nitella* according to Eq. (8.3) and added up, the sum still fell short of the plasmalemma conductance, g_p, as the following average figures show (μmho cm^{-2}):

g_K	g_{Na}	g_{Cl}	$g_K + g_{Na} + g_{Cl}$	g_p
7	1	(1)	9	21

Results from *Chara* showed a similar discrepancy. Several investigators believe that proton conductance will prove significant. However, there are reasons for believing that the fluxes (and therefore changes in fluxes with ψ_m—the partial ion conductance) are underestimated because of depletion and enhancement of concentration outside the plasmalemma. These effects were discussed in Chapter 7 in connection with 'electrogenic pumps'. It is apparent that a discontinuity in transport number at a surface may result in a local decrease or increase in concentration. Dewhurst (1960) has discussed this effect under the heading 'concentration polarisation'. If, in the cells under consideration, an inward flow of positive current is carried by K^+ through the plasmalemma but by Ca^{++} and Na^+ in the cell wall (owing to their preponderance as counterions), a depletion of K^+ will result just outside the membrane. The p.d. being K^+-sensitive, it will drift more negative (inside) and this is always observed to some extent in *Chara* during the prolonged passage of hyperpolarising currents (Barry and Hope, 1969 b). Conversely, a positive outward current should cause a drift towards increased depolarisation because of enhancement of K^+ just outside the plasmalemma. Such drifts are also observed. It is clear, at least for inward currents, that during such drifts the influx must decrease owing to falling K_o, even if it tends to increase owing to a rising value of $\psi_K - \psi_m$. Backflux during build-up of specific activity in the cell wall, during efflux experiments, was also noted by Walker and Hope (1969) as a further cause of underestimation of fluxes. Thus the 'non-independence' for K^+ so far found in plant cells is probably a lower limit.

8.6 CONCLUSIONS

Experiments with radioactive tracers have shown that there is a constant movement of ions into and out of cells. This traffic is described in terms of influxes and effluxes of ions across the cell membranes, which are apparently rate-limiting for radiotracer equilibration.

The influx and efflux of potassium have been shown to interact in squid axons and in *Chara* and *Nitella* membranes. The fluxes of potassium are thus not independent. This suggests that these ions do not cross membranes in a dilute solution, in which the only frictional opposition encountered would be expected to be with the membrane material itself.

We would be on the way to a complete description of fluxes, membrane conductance and potentials if the interactions between ions could be clarified.

Departures from independence are possibly due to fluxes of other ions or even of metabolic products and metabolites, according to Coster and George (1968). These interactions need not, but *may*, take place in pores or otherwise differentiated places in cell membranes.

Although the pore model mentioned in Sub-section 8.5.1 above has not found favour owing to its arbitrariness, calculations of the expected flux ratios do in fact agree with the direction and approximate magnitude of the observed deviations from Ussing's equation (Harris, 1960; Lea, 1963).

9

Metabolism and active transport

9.1 INTRODUCTION

In this chapter it is proposed to follow up the findings of earlier sections in which it was clearly indicated that many aspects of ionic movements or distributions need the intervention of 'active' mechanisms. We wish to know the extent to which active transport is found throughout plant and animal organs or cells, and the extent to which it is connected with a particular, common aspect of metabolism.

A conventional method of studying the connection between the metabolism on the one hand and ion fluxes on the other has been through the effects of metabolic inhibitors. A second method has been to correlate the level or rate of metabolism with the size of an ion flux or of the concentration ratio between the inside and outside of cells. These methods are open to criticism in some instances and experiments must be designed which allow more positive inferences to be made.

9.2 THE ACTIVE TRANSPORT OF SODIUM

9.2.1 The widespread occurrence of sodium transport

In Chapter 6 it was shown that in a number of systems a flux of sodium ions occurred against an electrochemical potential gradient, or occurred when the gradient was reduced to zero by short-circuiting the preparation. When the flux is between two aqueous media, it is difficult to see how the hypothesis of active sodium transport can be avoided. The phenomenon has been observed in a large number of biological systems in addition to the nerve, muscle and algal cells which were discussed in Chapter 6. Table 9.1 lists some further preparations in which an active sodium flux has been held to be involved in the ionic relations.

Table 9.1

Preparation	Animal or plant	Main evidence	Reference
Tubules of kidney	Rat	Net transport against electrochemical gradient	Giebisch (1964)
Cortex slices, kidney	Guinea-pig	Na^+ extruded against electrochemical gradient	Whittembury (1965)
Illium	Rabbit	Short-circuit current equal to Na flux	Schultz and Zalusky (1964)
Thallus	*Porphyra* (red alga)	Na efflux light- and CN^--dependent	Eppley (1958, 1959)
Red blood cells	Sheep	Effects of strophanthidin and concentration of K^+, etc.	Tosteson and Hoffman (1960)
RBC ghosts	Man	Dependence on metabolism Link with K influx Effect of strophanthidin	Hoffman (1962)
Roots or epicotyl	*Pisum* and *Avena*	Sodium below level predicted by potential and external concentration	Higinbotham, Etherton and Foster (1967)
Bladder	Toad (*Bufo*)	Short-circuit current equal to Na flux	Frazier, Dempsey and Leaf (1962)
Bladder	Turtle	Net Na^+ flux under short-circuit conditions: glycolysis involved	Klahr and Bricker (1965)
Gall-bladder	Rabbit, guinea-pig	Transport against electrochemical gradient	Diamond (1964)

9.2.2   Sodium efflux pumps and phosphorylation

The experiments of Hodgkin and Keynes with *Sepia* axons have been referred to several times (Chapter 8). In these and later experiments there was a very clear indication that active extrusion of sodium depended on oxidative metabolism: 0·2 mM DNP had the effect of decreasing the efflux of sodium by a factor of about 30; 1 mM NaCN and 3 mM NaN_3 had similar effects. Potassium influx was strongly affected at the same time. Mean fluxes in these experiments (Hodgkin and Keynes, 1955 a) were:

K	ϕ_i	15–30	ϕ_o	27	(control)
		2–3		33	(+ inhibitor)
Na	ϕ_i	23	ϕ_o	30–50	(control)
		15		1·5–5	(+ inhibitor)

In contrast to these results, Frazier and Keynes (1959) observed only a slow decline in the rate constant for sodium efflux in frog sartorius muscle when they added 2 mM CN^- + 5 mM iodoacetate. These inhibitors together were expected to slow down production of adenosine triphosphate (ATP) in both respiration and glycolysis. Possibly a store of ATP in the muscle sufficed for the energy needed to extrude sodium ions against an electrochemical gradient.

Some further important results were obtained by Caldwell et al. (1960 a, b) which point to cellular phosphorylation as being involved rather closely with sodium extrusion. In Loligo axons CN^- inhibition of efflux of Na^+ could be relieved temporarily by injecting organic phosphates into the axoplasm. Thus at about 10–20 mM in the axoplasm arginine phosphate was most effective and ATP almost as effective; phosphoenolpyruvate was less effective; and creatine phosphate, ineffective. ATP and arginine phosphate were ineffective on the outside. Brinley and Mullins (1967) made measurements of ATP consumption in dialysed axons of Loligo pealei during ATP-fuelled sodium extrusion and found a consumption rate of 43 pmol $cm^{-2} s^{-1}$; the sodium efflux averaged about 50 pmol $cm^{-2} s^{-1}$. The difficulties in estimating the efficiency of this use of energy were stressed.

This and other evidence from red blood cells suggested a link between some sorts of ion transport and reactions in cells or cell membranes involving phosphorylation and hydrolysis of adenosine phosphates, and led to the ready acceptance of the transport ATP-ase hypothesis. This will be considered in more detail later.

9.2.3   Coupling between sodium and potassium fluxes

Any active transport process must be governed by a condition of electroneutrality in the absence of an externally flowing current. That is, an efflux of sodium must be balanced by the influx of another cation or the efflux of an anion. If Na^+ were being removed from an ion exchange region, constancy of numbers of fixed charges might enforce a one-for-one replacement by whatever cations could most easily permeate—usually potassium. This seems to be observed sometimes (Glynn, 1957) but in other cells potassium influx is less than an associated active sodium efflux (Frazier and Leaf, 1963), or the time-courses of recovery to a high-potassium, low-sodium level in cells previously put in a low-K medium are different (Eppley, 1958).

9.2.4   Active fluxes in anaerobic conditions

In bladders from fresh-water turtles Klahr and Bricker (1965) found a fair correlation between anaerobic glycolysis (measured by lactate formation) and net sodium transport. The level of glycolysis depended on the presence of sodium in the Ringer's solution, since the rate dropped to 55% of control in choline Ringer's. The average level of ATP in the tissue did not change appreciably between the aerobic and anaerobic conditions.

In red blood cells from mammals the energy for active transport of sodium and potassium comes from glycolysis, but birds and reptiles have RBCs in which oxidative metabolism is necessary (Maizels, 1954). The distinction is usually made through the different effects of classes of inhibitors for the two types of metabolism—cyanide, azide and DNP on the one hand, and fluoride and iodo-acetate on the other.

9.3 TRANSPORT ATP-ASES

Some of the background has just been given that has led to belief in the involvement of ATP and, probably, of enzymes associated with its turnover and conversion. A particular ATP-ase was isolated from peripheral nerves by Skou (1957) which in several ways was suggestive of its direct involvement in active transport of the linked sodium–potassium sort: (a) the activity of the ATP-ase was dependent on Mg^{++}, K^+ and Na^+; (b) the ATP-ase had a high affinity for K^+ *in the presence of a high concentration of* Na^+; (c) the activation of the enzyme with K^+ and Na^+ occurred with ATP as a substrate but not with uridine or guanosine triphosphate; and (d) cardiac glycosides such as ouabain (g-strophanthin) inhibited that part of the ATP-ase activity stimulated by K^+ and Na^+.

In some instances there was quantitative agreement between the concentration-dependence of the ATP-ase activity (hydrolysis of ATP) and the concentration-dependence of active transport rate. Ouabain inhibited each of these functions at not very different concentrations. These and other aspects are reviewed by Skou (1965).

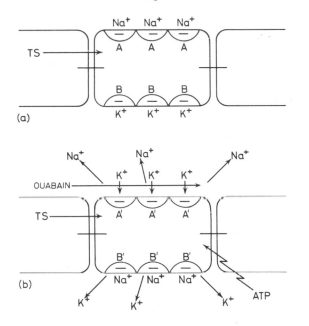

Fig. 9.1   Sodium–potassium-linked ATP-ase transport system (TS) according to Skou (1965): (a) and (b) represent different stages in the transport of potassium ions, originally outside, to the inside, and sodium ions, originally inside, to the outside. Stage (a) becomes stage (b) on adsorption and hydrolysis of an ATP molecule. Stage (b) may revert to stage (a) by a rotation of a sector of membrane or by virtue of the carrier sites being mobile. Ouabain is shown as preventing the adsorption of K^+ to exchange sites A' on the outside

It has been suggested that such an ATP-ase acts as part of an ion transport system, TS, along the following lines.

The deactivated form is shown in Fig. 9.1 (a) with sodium ions having just arrived from the inside, where they became bound to sites A preferential to Na^+. Three potassium ions (originally outside) are bound to three sites B which prefer K^+.

In Fig. 9.1 (b) the next stage of the transport is outlined. ATP, which is found to be active only on the inside, becomes bound to the TS and causes the sites A and B to change their properties. A changes from sodium-selective to potassium-selective, and B *vice versa*.

A convenient reversal of anionic field strength might be suggested to cause this change in selectivity (see Chapter 5, Section 5.3). Presumably, energy is needed to change the sites A and B to A', B'. Thus, hydrolysis, rather than merely adsorption, of ATP must take place at this stage. The TS then flips so that sites A' and B' are now on opposite sides. No energy seems to be needed here but it must be timed properly. Three sites are shown since about three Na^+ ions are transported per ATP hydrolysed in some experiments (Sen and Post, 1961).

Ouabain possibly acts by preventing K^+ occupying K^+-preferring sites on the outside (it does not work on the inside), or by displacing K^+ from them. Competitive inhibition is not involved, however. Schemes such as this even if little better than magic, at least inspire the imagination, and serve to summarise the correlations found. Opit and Charnock (1965) have elaborated the ATP-driven transport system somewhat.

A further hypothesis indicating how an ATP-ase could be connected with ion transport is that due to Mitchell (1966). The ATP-ase is within a membrane structure and coupled to an oxidation–reduction chain. Up to two protons may be translocated per ATP hydrolysed. The operation of this system is said to result in a gradient of protons across a membrane impermeable to them and in a potential difference as well. It is not at all clear how the proton gradient should be connected with a p.d. when the membrane in the model is supposedly impermeable to protons, except to cause an electrostatic charge on the membrane acting as a capacitor. If the membrane is in fact somewhat permeable to ions, then any p.d. would be a complex function of the gradients of all the ion species to which the membrane was at all permeable, through some equation such as (1.10). Finally the model offers the possibility of proton exchange for metal cations through 'exchange diffusion' pathways. Mitchell has recently elaborated on the more biophysical aspects of the 'chemiosmotic theory' in Vol. 2 (1969) of *Theoretical and experimental biophysics*.

In plant tissue a salt-stimulated ATP-ase corresponding to acid phosphatase has been isolated (see Atkinson and Polya, 1967). The enzyme is ouabain-insensitive and for this and other reasons it does not correspond to K^+, Na^+-stimulated ATP-ase from animal tissues.

9.4 LIGHT-DEPENDENT CHLORIDE TRANSPORT IN PLANT CELLS

There is very clear evidence that most of the chloride influx in Characean cells is dependent on continuing photosynthesis. The stimulation of influx in light is a widespread observation (dating from 1923—Hoagland and Davis). It was shown in Chapter 6 that chloride ions are about 200–250 mV away from electrochemical equilibrium in *Nitella* and *Chara*. This corresponds to energy expenditure at the rate of about 6000 cal mol^{-1} as Cl$^-$ is transported inwards.

The following table summarizes some of the effects of inhibitors on the influx of chloride. All the inhibitors have marked effects on some aspect of photosynthesis when this is examined in other systems: for example, in isolated chloroplasts. There is some doubt as to whether the same effects were operating in the intact cells used in the determination of fluxes of chloride. The work suffers from 'extrapolation' of this sort, which will no doubt shortly be rectified by making parallel biochemical studies.

In the meantime the data summarised in Table 9.2 allow certain generalisations to be made about the role of photosynthesis in chloride transport.

Influx of chloride decreases markedly when photosynthetic electron transport is reduced. MacRobbie (1965; 1966 a, b) proposes that it is the continuing process of net electron flow in photosystem II that is necessary. It is interesting that the influx very rarely falls below 0·1–0·5 pequiv. cm^{-2} s^{-1} even in prolonged dark periods. This dark influx may be an active one, dependent on respiration or glycolysis, or part of an exchange diffusion system. There is some indication of the latter in *C. corallina*.

Most of the evidence is consistent with MacRobbie's hypothesis, which has found support in a study of another green alga, *Hydrodictyon africanum* (Raven, 1967 a, b). However, since CCCP and phlorizin affect chloride transport and phlorizin, specifically, affects photosynthetic phosphorylation, this hypothesis may need some modification. The light-stimulated chloride influx in *Griffithsia* is DCMU-sensitive, as in the plants mentioned above, which, again, implicates the electron transport in photosystem II as being closely concerned with active transport of anions. The connection between photosynthetic processes occurring in a layer of chloroplasts and active transport at the plasmalemma or tonoplast is quite obscure at present.

Table 9.2 EFFECTS OF INHIBITORS ON ACTIVE INFLUX OF CHLORIDE IN
Nitella AND *Chara*

Inhibitor (conc.)	Influx(pequiv.cm^{-2}s^{-1})		Inhib./control (%) (when significantly different)	Reference
	Control (L)	+ Inhibitor		
Dark	3·2	0·23	7	A
DCMU (1) 1 μM	2·3	0·36	16	C
DCMU 1·3 μM	1·9	0·98, 1·05	52, 55	B
Far red light (2)	1·9	0·58	30	C
Imidazole 0·1 mM (3)	2·3	2·16	—	C
Imidazole 0·1 mM	1·15	1·58	137	B
CCCP (4) 5 μM	1·0	0·77	—	D
CCCP 2 μM	0·85	0·30	35	B
3 μM	1·91	0·3	16	B
10 μM	1·91	0·08 (cells not streaming	4	B
Paraquat (5) 0·1 mM	3·2	0·58	18	B
	1·75	1·59	—	B
	0·85	0·27	32	B
Phlorizin (6) 0·1 mM	1·91	0·94	49	B
	0·85	0·24	28	B
Azide (7) 0·5 mM	2·0	0·82	41	B

A, MacRobbie (1964), B, Coster and Hope (1968), C, MacRobbie (1965), D, MacRobbie (1966 a).
1. DCMU: Dichlorophenyl dimethylurea. Prevents electron flow from plastoquinone to quinone and cytochromes in photosynthetic schemes (Duysens, 1963).
2. Far red light: 705 < λ < 730 nm: System I but not System II operative in photosynthesis (ref. C).
3. Imidazole: Uncoupler of photosynthetic phosphorylation (p.p.) (see ref. C).
4. CCCP: Carbonyl cyanide m-chlorophenyl hydrazone. Uncouples p.p. from electron flow in photosynthesis (Nobel, 1967).
5. Paraquat: N,N′dimethyl-4,4′-dipyridylium dichloride. Competes for electrons with the normal acceptors.
6. Phlorizin: Specific inhibitor of p.p. (Nobel, 1967).
7. Azide: Inhibitor of cytochromes in the redox system of photosynthesis.

9.5 POTASSIUM AND SODIUM ACTIVE TRANSPORT IN PLANTS

Part of the influx of potassium in *Nitella*, *Chaetomorpha*, *Valonia* and *Hydrodictyon* is coupled to metabolism (Chapter 6). In the interpretation of the effects of inhibitors on fluxes of cations, however, caution must be used. In *Chara* potassium ions are close to being in electrochemical equilibrium. In *Nitella* ψ_K is more negative than ψ_m; thus, given equality of influx and efflux, it is necessary that some of the influx be active. In both these genera an effect of membrane potential on potassium influx can be obtained (Chapter 8) so that some of the influx is passive, the proportion varying with season or with time of storage after collection of plants from ponds.

Hence, when an inhibitor causes a lowered influx of K^+, it could be due to (a) a change in p.d. causing a change in $\psi_K - \psi_m$ and, hence, in ϕ_K, or (b) a change in membrane resistance upon which ϕ_K changes because of the relation $\phi_K = g_K(\psi_K - \psi_m)$, or (c) a change in the rate of some active transport process. Possibility (a) is sometimes examined (MacRobbie, 1966 a; Raven, 1967 a) but (b) rarely, conclusion (c) being then reached.

Effects of inhibitors on membrane resistance have been observed on a number of occasions. Hope, Simpson and Walker (1966) found that with *Nitella* and *Chara* cells dark conditions and 1 μM DCMU were similar in leading to an increased efflux of chloride (about 2 units) compared with light (0·5 units). In *Chara* DCMU may nevertheless cause an *increase* in the resistance of the plasmalemma from 8 to 50 kΩ cm². In *Chaetomorpha*, where Cl^- ions are not far from equilibrium, both influx and efflux were lowered considerably by addition of 5 μM CCCP.

The effects argue in favour of a link between membrane structure and metabolism which should repay study. However, allowing for reservations of this sort, it appears that active transport of cations is connected with photophosphorylation in green algae. In rare instances in plants, e.g. as discussed by Raven (1967 a), ouabain affects the influx of K^+ and the efflux of Na^+; the concentration needed is rather higher than in animals (1 mM in *Hydrodictyon*). In this plant also a degree of coupling between K^+ influx and Na^+ efflux was observed.

9.6 CONCLUSIONS

Cells are organised to affect the movement of certain ions in a direction opposite to that expected on the grounds of the established electrochemical potential gradient. Energy from some other cell function must be provided for this.

At present, only the vaguest ideas about the link between active transport and metabolic reactions have been formed, with one or two exceptions. The Na, K-stimulated ATP-ase, the properties of which were discussed in Section 9.3, has many aspects in common with the active transport of Na linked with that of K, in the way the ATP-ase is affected by ions and inhibitors. Thus, it seems likely that there is an intimate relationship between this particular enzyme and ion transport, *in vivo*. Several models suggesting modes of action of the ATP-ase in membranes have been described but many of the details are obscure.

Active chloride transport in certain algae is thought to be linked with so-called 'net electron flow' in photosynthetic reactions. Once again, future experiments must be relied upon to fill in the details of the connection.

10

Conclusions

10.1 SOME UNSCIENTIFIC GENERALISATIONS

Ion transport and a controlling function of membranes are both characteristic of most living cells. If a little teleology can be tolerated in the last chapter, it might be surmised that a high-potassium, low-sodium regime within cytoplasm is favourable for the efficient working of various enzyme systems. In addition, membranes have evolved in some cells which make use of the e.m.f. represented by the gradients of sodium and potassium across them. These excitable membranes are in a sense pulse generators in which current flows briefly when the membrane becomes transiently more permeable to sodium. Excitable membranes in animals are associated with transmission of nerve impulses and muscle contraction. In plants excitability appears to be associated with quick mechanical movements in the bizarre plants *Mimosa* and *Dionaea*. In Characean plants excitability seems to serve no particular function at all unless, being rather chloride-impermeable, the membrane leaks KCl in the action potential to prevent an explosion, after particularly active, active transport.

Cell membranes are not as impermeable as are some of the ultrathin, lipid films investigated (Chapter 3). Presumably, natural membranes must be able to pass readily gaseous molecules, water and metabolites. A limited permeability to environmental ions goes with this. Thus active removal of sodium ions, together with some anions, becomes necessary to prevent osmotic disorder, unless the membrane is surrounded by a rigid wall, or unless the cytoplasm has some structural rigidity. A one-for-one coupling of sodium efflux would do little to help the osmotic balance were it not for the additional factor of relative impermeability of the membrane to sodium ions. Thus a muscle fibre immersed in Ringer's solution is a double Donnan system: the sodium forming the indiffusible ions of the Ringer's solution; and protein or phospholipid charges, etc., the indiffusible (anions) of the sarcoplasm. Potassium and chloride ions form the common, diffusible ions in both phases. The imbibitional tendencies of the two Donnan phases tend to cancel out.

In vacuolated plant cells, as well as potassium enrichment of the cytoplasm, we find accumulation of ion pairs in the vacuole at a high osmotic potential compared with the environment. Even marine coenocytes have a turgor pressure of several atmospheres. This may be associated with a large difference between the volume of cells at mitosis compared with that at maturity; the osmotic potential for expansion is correlated with a steady plastic deformation and synthesis of cell walls. Also, the erect habit of plants goes with turgor pressure and with structural stiffening by cellulose.

10.2 FUTURE RESEARCH

We are barely emerging from the preliminary stages of investigating cells in relation to ions. Progress has been slow—understandably, in view of the great complexity of living systems. To obtain an idea of the sizes of the fluxes of ions and of the forces acting is a slow and tedious process. However, with the present body of knowledge and range of techniques it should be possible to decide between hypotheses more quickly. More collaboration between biochemists and biophysicists should prove fruitful. For example, the fractionation of cytoplasmic ion content between soluble cytoplasm and organelles should be feasible in density gradients of non-polar solvents. Also, one would wish that the effects of metabolic inhibitors could be studied more frequently using whole cells rather than subcellular organelles.

The testing of models for some aspect of membrane function is expected to become easier through the use of computers, and useful in so far as the experimentalist keeps providing unequivocal data. One fully expects that theoretical flux ratios will soon be worked out for various shapes of pores and slits, charged or uncharged.

In the search for ion pumps a challenging hypothesis has emerged. This is the concept that active transport of ions against an electrochemical gradient is a reflection of 'entrainment' between the ions and fluxes of substances such as metabolic substrates going into the cell and metabolic products emerging (Chapter 2).

In this view discrimination between sodium and potassium

would reside in a greater friction between potassium ions and influxing molecules X (entering the cell down a gradient for X). Effluxing molecules Y might interact more with sodium ions tending to move inwards down the electrochemical gradient for Na^+. This is an attractive hypothesis and should be tested. The effects of inhibitors would enter the scheme naturally through their effects on the gradients of X and Y.

This book has made frequent mention of sodium, potassium and chloride ions, and rather neglected at least two other ion species, namely calcium and hydrogen. (Or is it hydroxonium? One can't tell with membranes.) Present indications are that these two species have a controlling influence on the more populous ions. We must use all our ingenuity to develop means to detect movements of protons, as, unfortunately, there is no convenient radioactive tracer for them.

This book will have served its purpose if it has conveyed a little of the fascination of experimental work with cells and electrolytes. There was some years ago no very good *a priori* reason why giant cells should serve as examples of more usual cellular life. At present, however, I feel there is more justification for extrapolation. Processes and principles observed in the large cells have increasingly been found to be similar in smaller ones. I refer to membrane potentials and resistance, in roots, coleoptiles, moss thallus, stem tissue, fungi and multicellular water plants as well as in coenocytes. Active transport of sodium and potassium has similarities to that in axons in cells from blood, kidney tubules, frog skin and bladder, plant coenocytes and roots, muscle fibres and bacteria.

May the squid, barnacles and giant algae of the oceans prosper.

References

ANDREOLI, T. E., BANGHAM, J. A. and TOSTESON, D. C. (1967). The formation and properties of thin lipid membranes from HK and LK sheep red cell lipids. *J. gen. Physiol.* **50** (6, 1), 1729

ANDREOLI, T. E., TIEFFENBERG, M. and TOSTESON, D. C. (1967). The effect of valinomycin on the ionic permeability of thin lipid membranes. *J. gen. Physiol.* **50** (11), 2527

ATKINSON, M. R., FINDLAY, G. P., HOPE, A. B., PITMAN, M. G., SADDLER, H. D. W. and WEST, K. R. (1967). Salt regulation in the mangroves *Rhizophora mucronata* Lam. and *Aegialitis annulata* R. Br. *Aust. J. biol. Sci.* **20**, 289

ATKINSON, M. R. and POLYA, G. (1967). Salt stimulated adenosine triphosphatases from carrot, beet and *Chara australis. Aust. J. biol. Sci.* **20**, 1069

BAKER, P. F., HODGKIN, A. L. and SHAW, T. I. (1961). Replacement of the protoplasm of a giant nerve fibre with artificial solutions. *Nature, Lond.* **190**, 885

BARR, C. E. (1965). Na and K fluxes in *Nitella clavata. J. gen. Physiol.* **49** (2), 181

BARRY, P. H. (1967). Ph.D. Thesis, University of Sydney

BARRY, P. H. and HOPE, A. B. (1969 a). Electroosmosis in membranes: effects of unstirred layers. I. Theory. *Biophys. J.* **9** (5), 700

BARRY, P. H. and HOPE, A. B. (1969 b). Electroosmosis in membranes: effects of unstirred layers. II. Experimental. *Biophys. J.* **9** (5), 729

BLINKS, L. R. (1930). The direct current resistance of *Valonia. J. gen. Physiol.* **13** (3), 361

BLOUNT, R. W. and LEVEDAHL, B. H. (1960). Active sodium and chloride transport in the single-celled alga *Halicystis ovalis. Acta Physiol. scand.* **49**, 1

BRADLEY, J. and WILLIAMS, E. J. (1967). Chloride electrochemical potentials and membrane resistances in *Nitella translucens. J. exp. Bot.* **18**, 241

BRANTON, D. (1966). Fracture faces of frozen membranes. *Proc. natn Acad. Sci. U.S.A.* **55** (5), 1048

BRIGGS, G. E. (1962). Membrane potential difference in *Chara australis. Proc. R. Soc.* B **156**, 573

BRIGGS, G. E. (1967). Electro-osmosis in *Nitella. Proc. R. Soc. B* **168**, 22

BRIGGS, G. E., HOPE, A. B. and ROBERTSON, R. N. (1961). *Electrolytes and plant cells*, Blackwell Scientific Publications, Oxford

BRINLEY, F. J. and MULLINS, L. J. (1967). Sodium extrusion by internally dialysed squid axons. *J. gen. Physiol.* **50** (10), 2303

CALDWELL, P. C., HODGKIN, A. L., KEYNES, R. D. and SHAW, T. I. (1960 a). The effects of injecting 'energy-rich' phosphate compounds on the active transport of ions in the giant axons of *Loligo. J. Physiol., Lond.* **152**, 561

CALDWELL, P. C., HODGKIN, A. L., KEYNES, R. D. and SHAW, T. I. (1960 b). Partial inhibition of the active transport of cations in the giant axons of *Loligo*. *J. Physiol.* **152**, 591

CASS, A. and FINKELSTEIN, A. (1967). Water permeability of thin lipid membranes. *J. gen. Physiol.* **50** (6, 1), 1765

COLE, K. S. (1962). The advance of electrical models for cells and axons. *Biophys. J.* **2** (2, 2), 101

COLE, K. S. (1965). Electro-diffusion models for the membrane of the squid giant axon. *Physiol. Rev.* **45**, 340

COLE, K. S. and HODGKIN, A. L. (1939). Membrane and protoplasm resistance in the squid giant axon. *J. gen. Physiol.* **22**, 671

COPE, F. W. (1967). NMR evidence for complexing of Na⁺ in muscle, kidney and brain, and by actomyosin. The relation of cellular complexing of Na⁺ to water structure and to transport kinetics. *J. gen. Physiol.* **50** (5), 1353

COSTER, H. G. L. (1965). A quantitative analysis of the voltage-current relationships of fixed charge membranes and the associated property of the 'punch-through'. *Biophys. J.* **5** (5), 669

COSTER, H. G. L. (1966). Chloride of cells of *Chara australis*. *Aust. J. biol. Sci.* **19**, 545

COSTER, H. G. L. and GEORGE, P. (1968). A thermodynamic analysis of fluxes and flux-ratios in biological membranes. *Biophys. J.* **8** (4), 457

COSTER, H. G. L. and HOPE, A. B. (1968). Ionic relations of cells of *Chara australis*. XI. Chloride fluxes. *Aust. J. biol. Sci.* **21**, 243

CRANK, J. (1956). *The mathematics of diffusion*, Clarendon Press, Oxford

DAINTY, J. (1963). Water relations of plant cells. In: *Advances in Botanical Research*, Ed. R. D. Preston, Vol. I, Academic Press, London

DAINTY, J. and GINZBURG, B. Z. (1964). The measurement of hydraulic conductivity (osmotic permeability to water) of internodal characean cells by means of transcellular osmosis. *Biochim. biophys. Acta*. **79**, 102

DAINTY, J. and HOPE, A. B. (1959). Ionic relations of cells of *Chara australis*. I. Ion exchange in the cell wall. *Aust. J. biol. Sci.* **12**, 395

DAINTY, J. and HOPE, A. B. (1961). The electric double layer and the Donnan equilibrium in relation to plant cell walls. *Aust. J. biol. Sci.* **14**, 541

DANIELLI, J. F. and DAVSON, H. (1952). In: *Permeability of natural membranes* by H. DAVSON and J. F. DANIELLI, Cambridge University Press

DEAN, R. B., CURTIS, H. J. and COLE, K. S. (1940). Impedance of bimolecular films. *Science, N.Y.* **91**, 50

DEGROOT, S. R. and MAZUR, P. (1962). *Non-equilibrium thermodynamics*. North-Holland, Amsterdam

DENBIGH, K. G. (1951). *The thermodynamics of the steady state*. Methuen, London

DESPIC, A. and HILLS, G. J. (1956). Electro-osmosis in charged membranes. The determination of primary solvation numbers. *Discuss. Faraday Soc.* **21**, 150

DEWHURST, D. J. (1960). Concentration polarisation in plane membrane-solution systems. *Trans. Faraday Soc.* **56** (1), 599

DIAMOND, J. M. (1962). The mechanism of water transport by the gall bladder. *J. Physiol.* **161**, 503

DIAMOND, J. M. (1964). The mechanism of isotonic water transport. *J. gen. Physiol.* **48** (1), 15

DIAMOND, J. M. (1966). A rapid method for determining voltage-concentration relations across membranes. *J. Physiol.* **183**, 83

DIAMOND, J. M. and TORMEY, J. McD. (1966). Studies on the structural basis of water transport across epithelial membranes. *Fedn Proc. Fedn Am. Socs exp. Biol.* **25**, 1458

DIAMOND, J. M. and WRIGHT, E. M. (1969). Biological membranes: the physical basis of ion and non-electrolyte selectivity. *Ann. Rev. Physiol.* **31**, 581

DODD, W. A., PITMAN, M. G. and WEST, K. R. (1966). Sodium and potassium transport in the marine alga *Chaetomorpha darwinii*. *Aust. J. biol. Sci.* **19**, 341

DUYSENS, L. N. M. (1963). In: *Photosynthesis mechanisms in green plants*, Publication 1145 of National Academy of Sciences (Netherlands) National Research Council

EISENMAN, G. (1960). On the elementary atomic origin of equilibrium ionic specificity. In: *Symposium on membrane transport and metabolism*, Academic Press, New York

EISENMAN, G. (1962). Cation selective glass electrodes and their mode of operation. *Biophys. J.* **2** (2, 2), 259

EISENMAN, G. (1963). The influence of Na, K, Li, Rb, and Cs on cellular potentials and related phenomena. *Bulletin del Instituto de Estudios Medicos y Biologicos (Mexico)* **XXI** (2), 155

EPPLEY, R. W. (1958). Potassium-dependent sodium extrusion by cells of *Porphyra perforata*, a red marine alga. *J. gen. Physiol.* **42** (2), 281

EPPLEY, R. W. (1959). Potassium accumulation and sodium efflux by *Porphyra perforata* tissues in lithium and magnesium sea water. *J. gen. Physiol.* **43** (1), 29

FENSOM, D. S. and DAINTY, J. (1963). Electro-osmosis in *Nitella*. *Can. J. Bot.* **41**, 685

FINDLAY, G. P. and HOPE, A. B. (1964). Ionic relations of cells of *Chara australis*. VII. The separate electrical characteristics of the plasmalemma and tonoplast. *Aust. J. biol. Sci.* **17**, 66

FINDLAY, G. P., HOPE, A. B. and WILLIAMS, E. J. (1969). Ionic relations of marine algae, I. *Griffithsia*: Membrane electrical properties. *Aust. J. biol. Sci.* **22**, 1163

FINKLESTEIN, A. and CASS, A. (1968). Permeability and electrical properties of thin lipid membranes. *J. gen. Physiol.* **52** (1, 2), 145s

FRAZIER, H. S., DEMPSEY, E. F. and LEAF, A. (1962). Movement of sodium across the mucosal surface of the isolated toad bladder and its modification by vasopressin. *J. gen. Physiol.* **45** (3), 529

FRAZIER, H. S. and KEYNES, R. D. (1959). The effect of metabolic inhibitors on the sodium fluxes in sodium-loaded frog sartorius muscle. *J. Physiol.* **148**, 362

FRAZIER, H. S. and LEAF, A. (1963). The electrical characteristics of active sodium transport in the toad bladder. *J. gen. Physiol.* **46** (3), 491

FUJITA, H. and GOSTING, L. J. (1960). The new procedure for calculating the four diffusion coefficients of three component systems from Guoy diffusiometer data. *J. phys. Chem., Ithaca* **64**, 1256

GIEBISCH, G. (1964). Measurements of electrical potential differences on single nephrons of the perfused *Necturus* kidney. *J. gen. Physiol.* **44** (4), 659

GINZBURG, B. Z. and KATCHALSKY, A. (1963). The frictional coefficients of the flows of non-electrolytes through artificial membranes. *J. gen. Physiol.* **47** (2), 403

GIRARDIER, L., RUEBEN, J. P., BRANDT, P. W. and GRUNDFEST, H. (1963). Evidence for anion-permselective membrane in crayfish muscle fibres and its possible role in excitation-contraction coupling. *J. gen. Physiol.* **47** (1), 189

GLYNN, I. M. (1957). The ion permeability of the red cell membrane. *Prog. Biophys. biophys. Chem.* **8**, 241

GOLDMAN, D. E. (1943). Potential, impedance and rectification in membranes. *J. gen. Physiol.* **27**, 37

GRAHAM, J. and GERARD, R. W. (1946). Membrane potentials and excitation of impaled single muscle fibres. *J. cell. comp. Physiol.* **28**, 99

GREENHAM, C. G. (1966). The relative electrical resistances of the plasmalemma and tonoplast in higher plants. *Planta* **69**, 150

GUGGENHEIM, E. A. (1929). The conception of electrical potential between two phases and the individual activities of ions. *J. phys. Chem.* **33**, 842

GUTKNECHT, J. (1966). Sodium, potassium, and chloride transport and membrane potentials in *Valonia ventricosa*. *Biol. Bull.* **130**, 331

GUTKNECHT, J. (1967). Ion fluxes and short-circuit current in internally perfused cells of *Valonia ventricosa*. *J. gen. Physiol.* **50** (7), 1821

GUTKNECHT, J. and DAINTY, J. (1968). Ionic relations of marine algae. *Oceanogr. mar. Biol. Ann. Rev.* **6**, 163

HANAI, T., HAYDON, D. A. and REDWOOD, W. R. (1966). The water permeability of artificial bimolecular leaflets: a comparison of radio-tracer and osmotic methods. *Ann. N.Y. Acad. Sci.* **137** (2), 731

HANAI, T., HAYDON, D. A. and TAYLOR, J. (1964). An investigation by electrical methods of lecithin-in-hydrocarbon films in aqueous solutions. *Proc. R. Soc. Lond. A* **281**, 377

HARRIS, E. J. (1960). *Transport and accumulation in biological systems*, 2nd edn, Butterworths, London

HIGINBOTHAM, N., ETHERTON, B. and FOSTER, R. J. (1967). Mineral ion contents and cell transmembrane electropotentials of pea and oat seedling tissue. *Plant Physiol.* **42**, 37

HIGINBOTHAM, N., HOPE, A. B. and FINDLAY, G. P. (1964). Electrical resistance of cell membranes of *Avena* coleoptiles. *Science, N.Y.* **143**, 1448

HINKE, J. A. M. (1961). The measurement of sodium and potassium activities in the squid axon by means of cation-selective glass micro-electrodes. *J. Physiol.* **156**, 314

HOAGLAND, D. R. and DAVIS, A. R. (1923). Further experiments on the absorption of ions by plants, including observations on the effect of light. *J. gen. Physiol.* **6**, 47

HODGKIN, A. L. (1947). Membrane resistance of nerve. *J. Physiol.* **106**, 305

HODGKIN, A. L. (1951). The ionic basis of electrical activity in nerve and muscle. *Biol. Rev.* **26**, 339

HODGKIN, A. L. (1964). *The conduction of the nervous impulse*, Liverpool University Press

HODGKIN, A. L. and HOROWICZ, P. (1959 a). The influence of potassium and chloride ions on the membrane potential of single muscle fibres. *J. Physiol.* **148**, 127

HODGKIN, A. L. and HOROWICZ, P. (1959 b). Movements of Na and K in single muscle fibres. *J. Physiol.* **145**, 405

HODGKIN, A. L. and HUXLEY, A. F. (1952). Currents carried by sodium and potassium ions through the membrane of the giant axon of *Loligo*. *J. Physiol.* **116**, 449

HODGKIN, A. L. and HUXLEY, A. F. (1953). Movement of radioactive potassium and membrane current in a giant axon. *J. Physiol.* **121**, 403

HODGKIN, A. L. and KEYNES, R. D. (1953). The mobility and diffusion coefficient of potassium in giant axons from *Sepia*. *J. Physiol.* **119**, 513

HODGKIN, A. L. and KEYNES, R. D. (1955 a). Active transport of cations in giant axons from *Sepia* and *Loligo*. *J. Physiol.* **128**, 28

HODGKIN, A. L. and KEYNES, R. D. (1955 b). The potassium permeability of a giant nerve fibre. *J. Physiol.* **128**, 61

HOFFMAN, J. F. (1962). The active transport of sodium by ghosts of human red blood cells. *J. gen. Physiol.* **45** (5), 837

HOPE, A. B. (1956). The electric properties of plant cell membranes. I. The electric capacitance of suspensions of mitochondria, chloroplasts and *Chlorella* sp. *Aust. J. biol. Sci.* **9**, 53

HOPE, A. B. (1963). Ionic relations of cells of *Chara australis*. VI. Fluxes of potassium. *Aust. J. biol. Sci.* **16**, 429

HOPE, A. B. (1965). Ionic relations of cells of *Chara australis*. X. Effects of bicarbonate ions on electrical properties. *Aust. J. biol. Sci.* **18**, 789

HOPE, A. B., SIMPSON, A. and WALKER, N. A. (1966). The efflux of chloride from cells of *Nitella* and *Chara. Aust. J. biol. Sci.* **19**, 355

HOPE, A. B. and WALKER, N. A. (1960). Ionic relations of cells of *Chara australis*. III. Vacular fluxes of sodium. *Aust. J. biol. Sci.* **13**, 277

HOPE, A. B. and WALKER, N. A. (1961). Ionic relations of cells of *Chara australis*. IV. Membrane potential differences and resistances. *Aust. J. biol. Sci.* **14**, 26

HOPE, A. B. and WALKER, N. A. (1965). The effect of membrane potential upon ionic fluxes in cells of *Nitella translucens. J. Physiol.* **22** (P), 24

HOSHIKO, T. and LINDLEY, B. D. (1964). The relationship of Ussing's flux-ratio equation to the thermodynamic description of membrane permeability. *Biochim. biophys. Acta* **79**, 301

KARREMAN, G. and EISENMAN, G. (1952). Electrical potentials and ionic fluxes in ion exchangers: I. '*n* Type' non-ideal systems with zero current. *Bull. math. Biophys.* **24**, 413

KATCHALSKY, A. and CURRAN, P. F. (1965). *Non-equilibrium thermodynamics in biophysics*, Harvard University Press

KEDEM, O. (1961). In: *Symposium on membrane transport and metabolism.* p. 87, Academic Press, New York

KEDEM, O. and ESSIG, A. (1965). Isotope flows and flux ratios in biological membranes. *J. gen. Physiol.* **48** (6), 1047

KEDEM, O. and KATCHALSKY, A. (1961). A physical interpretation of the phenomenological coefficients of membrane permeability. *J. gen. Physiol.* **45**, 143

KEDEM, O. and KATCHALSKY, A. (1963). Permeability of composite membranes. Part I. Electric current, volume flow and flow of solute through membranes. *Trans. Faraday Soc.* **59**, 1918

KISHIMOTO, U. and TAZAWA, M. (1965). Ionic composition of the cytoplasm of *Nitella flexilis. Pl. Cell Physiol., Tokyo* **6**, 507

KLAHR, S. and BRICKER, N. S. (1965). Energetics of anaerobic sodium transport by the fresh water turtle bladder. *J. gen. Physiol.* **48** (4), 543

KOBATAKE, Y., TAKEGUCHI, N., TOYOSHIMA, Y. and FUJITA, H. (1965). Studies of membrane phenomena. I. Membrane potential. *J. phys. Chem.* **69** (3), 3981

KOEFOED-JOHNSEN, V., LEVI, H. and USSING, H. H. (1952). The mode of passage of chloride ions through the isolated frog skin. *Acta. Physiol. scand.* **25**, 150

LEA, E. J. A. (1963). Permeation through long narrow pores. *J. theoret. Biol.* **5**, 102

LEV, A. A. (1964). Determination of the activity and activity coefficients of potassium and sodium ions in frog muscle fibres by means of cation-sensitive glass microelectrodes. *Biofizika* **9** (6), 686

LEV, A. A. and BUZHINSKI, E. P. (1967). Cation specificity of model bimolecular phospholipid membranes with exposure to valinomycin. *Cytology (USSR)* **9**, 102

LING, G. N. (1962). *A physical theory of the living state,* Blaisdell, New York

LING, G. N. (1965). The physical state of water in living cell and model systems. In: Forms of water in biologic systems. *Ann. N.Y. Acad. Sci.* **125** (2), 401

LING, G. N. (1966). Cell membrane and cell permeability. In: Biological membranes: Recent progress. *Ann. N.Y. Acad. Sci.* **137** (2), 837

LOEWENSTEIN, W. R. and KANNO, G. (1963). The electric conductance and the membrane potential of some cell nuclei. *J. Cell. Biol.* **16**, 421

LOEWENSTEIN, W. R. and KANNO, G. (1964). Studies on an epithelial (gland) cell junction. I. Modifications of surface membrane permeability. *J. Cell. Biol.* **22**, 565

LOEWENSTEIN, W. R. and KANNO, G. (1966). Lack of intercellular communication between cancer cells. *Nature, Lond.* **209**, 1248

LUCY, J. A. (1964). Globular lipid micelles and cell membranes. *J. theoret. Biol.* **7** (2), 360

LUND, E. J. and collaborators (1947). *Bioelectric fields and growth*, University of Texas Press, Austin

MACKAY, D. and MEARES, P. (1959). The electrical conductivity and electro-osmotic permeability of a cation-exchange resin. *Trans. Faraday Soc.* **55**, 1221

MACROBBIE, E. A. C. (1962). Ionic relations of *Nitella translucens. J. gen. Physiol.* **45** (5), 861

MACROBBIE, E. A. C. (1964). Factors affecting the fluxes of potassium and chloride ions in *Nitella translucens. J. gen. Physiol.* **47** (5), 859

MACROBBIE, E. A. C. (1965). The nature of the coupling between light energy and active ion transport in *Nitella translucens. Biochim. biophys. Acta* **94**, 64

MACROBBIE, E. A. C. (1966 a). Metabolic effects on ion fluxes in *Nitella translucens.* I. Active transport. *Aust. J. biol. Sci.* **19**, 363

MACROBBIE, E. A. C. (1966 b). Metabolic effects on ion fluxes in *Nitella translucens.* II. Tonoplast fluxes. *Aust. J. biol. Sci.* **19**, 371

MACROBBIE, E. A. C. (1969). Ion fluxes to the vacuole of *Nitella translucens. J. exp. Bot.* **20**, 236

MACROBBIE, E. A. C. and DAINTY, J. (1958). Ion transport in *Nitellopsis obtusa. J. gen. Physiol.* **42** (2), 335

MACKIE, J. S. and MEARES, P. (1955). The sorption of electrolytes by a cation-exchange resin membrane. *Proc. R. Soc. A* **232**, 485

MAIZELS, M. (1954). Active cation transport in erythrocytes. *Symp. Soc. exp. Biol.* **8**, 202

MEARES, P. (1959). The fluxes of sodium and chloride ions across a cation-exchange resin membrane. Part 3. The application of irreversible thermodynamics. *Trans. Faraday Soc.* **55**, 1970

MEARES, P. and USSING, H. H. (1959). The fluxes of sodium and chloride ions across a cation-exchange resin membrane. Part 1. Effect of a concentration gradient. *Trans. Faraday Soc.* **55**, 142

MITCHELL, P. (1966). Chemiosmotic coupling in oxidative and photosynthetic phosphorylation. *Biol. Rev.* **41**, 445

MOOR, H. and MÜHLETHALER, K. (1963). Fine structure in frozen-etched yeast cells. *J. Cell. Biol.* **17** (3), 609

MUELLER, P., RUDIN, D. O., TI TIEN, H. and WESCOTT, W. C. (1963). Methods for the formation of single bimolecular lipid membranes in aqueuous solution. *J. phys. Chem.* **67** (1), 534

MUELLER, P. and RUDIN, D. O. (1967). Action potential phenomena in experimental bimolecular lipid membranes. *Nature, Lond.* **213**, 603

MÜHLETHALER, K. (1966). The ultrastructure of the plastid lamellae. In: *Biochemistry of chloroplasts.* Vol. 1, Academic Press, New York

MÜHLETHALER, K., MOOR, H. and SZARKOWSKI, J. W. (1965). The ultrastructure of the chloroplast lamellae. *Planta* **67**, 305

NAGAI, R. and KISHIMOTO, U. (1964). Cell wall potential in *Nitella. Pl. Cell Physiol.,* Tokyo **5**, 21

NOBEL, P. S. (1967). Calcium uptake, ATP ase and photophosphorylation by chloroplasts *in vitro. Nature, Lond.* **214**, 875

ONSAGER, L. (1931). Reciprocal relations in irreversible processes. I. *Phys. Rev.* **37**, 405; Reciprocal relations in irreversible processes. II. *Phys. Rev.* **38** (2), 2265

OPIT, L. J. and CHARNOCK, J. S. (1965). A molecular model for a sodium pump. *Nature, Lond.* **208**, 471

PAGANELLI, C. V. and SOLOMON, A. K. (1957). The rate of exchange of tritiated

water across the human red cell membrane. *J. gen. Physiol.* **41**, 259
PALLAGHY, C. K. and SCOTT, B. I. H. (1969). The electrochemical state of broad bean roots. II. Potassium kinetics in excised root tissue. *Aust. J. biol. Sci.* **22** (3), 585
PAULY, H., PACKER, L. and SCHWAN, H. P. (1960). Electrical properties of mitochondrical membranes. *J. biophys. biochem. Cytol.* **7**, 589
PIDOT, A. L. and DIAMOND, J. M. (1964). Streaming potentials in a biological membrane. *Nature, Lond.* **201**, 701
RAVEN, J. A. (1967 a). Ion transport in *Hydrodictyon africanum*. *J. gen. Physiol.* **50** (6), **1607**
RAVEN, J. A. (1967 b). Light stimulation of active transport in *Hydrodictyon africanum*. *J. gen. Physiol.* **50** (6), 1627
ROBINSON, R. A. and STOKES, R. H. (1955). *Electrolyte solutions,* Butterworth's London
ROSENBERG, S. A. (1969). A computer evaluation of equations for predicting the potential across biological membranes. *Biophys. J.* **9** (4), 500
SANDBLOM, J. P. and EISENMAN, G. (1967). Membrane potentials at zero current. The significance of a constant ionic permeability ratio. *Biophys. J.* **7**, 217
SCHULTZ, S. G. and ZALUSKY, R. (1964). Ion transport in isolated rabbit ileum. I. Short circuit current and Na fluxes. *J. gen. Physiol.* **47** (3), 567
SCHWAN, H. P. and COLE, K. S. (1960). Bioelectricity: Alternating current admittance of cells and tissues. In: *Medical physics.* Ed. O. GLASSEN, Vol. III, Year Book Publishers, Chicago
SEN, A. K. and POST, R. L. (1961). Stoichiometry of active Na $^+$ and K $^+$ transport to energy rich phosphate breakdown in human erythrocytes. *Fedn. Proc. Fedn. Am. Socs. exp. Biol.* **20**, 138
SJODIN, R. A. and HENDERSON, E. G. (1964). Tracer and non-tracer potassium fluxes in frog sartorius muscle and the kinetics of net potassium movement. *J. gen. Physiol.* **47** (4), 605
SKOU, J. C. (1957). The influence of some cations on an adenosinetriphosphatase from peripheral nerves. *Biochem. biophys. Acta* **23**, 394
SKOU, J. C. (1965). Enzymatic basis for active transport of Na $^+$ and K $^+$ across cell membrane. *Physiol. Rev.* **45**, 596
SLAYMAN, C. L. (1965). Electrical properties of *Neurospora crassa.* Respiration and the intracellular potential. *J. gen. Physiol.* **49** (1, 1), 93
SPANNER, D. C. (1964). *Introduction to thermodynamics,* Academic Press, New York
SPANSWICK, R. M., STOLAREK, J. and WILLIAMS, E. J., (1967). The membrane potential of *Nitella translucens. J. exp. Bot.* **18**, 1
SPANSWICK, R. M. and WILLIAMS, E. J. (1964). Electrical potentials and Na, K and Cl concentrations in the vacuole and cytoplasm of *Nitella translucens. J. exp. Bot.* **15**, 193
SPANSWICK, R. M. and WILLIAMS, E. J. (1965). Ca fluxes and membrane potentials in *Nitella translucens. J. exp. Bot.* **16**, 463
SPIEGLER, K. S. (1958). Transport processes in ionic membranes. *Trans. Faraday Soc.* **54**, 1408
STAVERMAN, A. J. (1952). Non-equilibrium thermodynamics of membrane processes. *Trans. Faraday Soc.* **48**, 176
STEIN, W. D. and DANIELLI, J. F. (1956). Structure and function in red cell permeability. *Discuss. Faraday Soc.* **21**, 238
STICKHOLM, A. and WALLIN, B. G. (1967). Relative ion permeabilities in the crayfish giant axon determined from rapid external ion changes. *J. gen. Physiol.* **50** (7), 1929
TAKAGA, M., AZUMA, K. and KISHIMOTO, U. (1965). A new method for the formation of bilayer membranes in aqueous solution. *Ann. Rep. biol. Works,* Osaka Univ.

13, 107

TAZAWA, M. and KAMIYA, N. (1966). Water permeability of a Characean internodal cell with special reference to its polarity. *Aust. J. biol. Sci.* **19**, 399

TEORELL, T. (1949). Membrane electrophoresis in relation to bio-electrical polarisation effects. *Arch. Sci. physiol.* **3**, 205

THOMPSON, T. E. and HUANG, C. (1966). The water permeability of lipid bilayer membranes. *Ann. N.Y. Acad. Sci.* **137** (2), 740

TOSTESON, D. C. and HOFFMAN, J. F. (1960). Regulation of cell volume by active transport in high and low potassium sheep red cells. *J. gen. Physiol.* **44** (1), 169

TROSHIN, A. S. (1960). Concerning an article by L. M. Chailakhian: Modern concepts of the nature of the resting potential. *Biophysics* (transl. Russian *Biofizika*) **5**, 104

TYLER, A., MONROY, A., KAO, C. Y. and GRUNDFEST, H. (1956). Membrane potential and resistance of the star fish egg before and after fertilisation. *Biol. Bull.* **111**, 153

UMRATH, K. (1930). Untersuchungen über Plasma und Plasmaströmung an Characeen. IV. Potentialmessungen an *Nitella mucronata* mit besonderer Berücksichtigung der Erregungserscheinung. *Proptoplasma* **9**, 576

USSING, H. H. (1949). The distinction by means of tracers between active transport and diffusion. *Acta Physiol. scand.* **19**, 43

USSING, H. H. (1965). *Transport of electrolytes and water across epithelia.* The Harvey Lectures Series 59, Academic Press, New York

USSING, H. H. and ZERAHN, K. (1951). Active transport of sodium as the source of the electric current in the short-circuited isolated frog skin. *Acta Physiol. scand.* **23**, 111

VAN ZUTPHEN, H., VAN DEENAN, L. L. M. and KINSKY, S. C. (1966). The action of polyene antibiotics on bilayer lipid membranes. *Biochem. biophys. Res. Commun.* **22**, 393

VOROBIEV, L. N. (1967). Potassium ion activity in the cytoplasm and the vacuole of cells of *Chara* and *Griffithsia*. *Nature, Lond.* **216** (5122), 1325

WALKER, N. A. (1960). The electric resistance of the cell membranes in a *Chara* and a *Nitella* species. *Aust. J. biol. Sci.* **13**, 468

WALKER, N. A. and Hope, A. B. (1969). Membrane fluxes and electrical conductance in Characean cells. *Aust. J. biol. Sci.* **22**, 1179

WHITTAM, R. and GUINNEBAULT, M. (1959). The efflux of potassium from electroplaques of electric eels. *J. gen. Physiol.* **43** (6, 1), 1171

WHITTEMBURY, G. (1965). Sodium extrusion and potassium uptake in guinea pig kidney cortex slices. *J. gen. Physiol.* **48** (4), 669

WILLIAMS, E. J., JOHNSTON, R. J. and DAINTY, J. (1964). The electrical resistance and capacitance of the membranes of Nitella translucens. *J. exp. Bot.* **15**, 1

Index

Active transport in *Nitella,* 63
  and flux ratio criterion, 67
  and Nernst criterion, 63
  and short-circuit technique, 68
ATP-ase, 102 ff
Avena membrane resistance, 73

Boltzmann equation, 9

Cellulose membrane, 39
  frictional coefficients in, 40
Chaetomorpha darwinii, 64
  ion fluxes, 93
Chara, 52
  active transport in, 64
  chloride transport, 105
  electro-osmosis in, 82
  K flux and p.d., 96
  membrane resistance, 73, 76
  punch-through in, 79
  rectification, 77
Characean cell, typical fluxes, 91
Compartments, animal cells, 13
  in models, 13, 16
  plant cells, 16
Conductance at Nernst potential, 12, 74
Conductance coefficients (phenomenological), 22
Coupled Na, K transport, 103
Crayfish, *see Procambarus clarkii*
Cuttlefish, *see Sepia officinalis,* giant
  axons from

Diffusion, 1
Drosophila, junctional resistance, 77

Electrochemical potential, 3
  gradient, 3

Electrogenic effects, 65
Electro-osmosis, 26, 29, 82
  in *Chara,* 81
  table, 82
Equilibrium potential, *see* Nernst
  potential

Flux of ions, 1
  and conductance, 12, 74
  net, 1, 6
  ratio, 9, 10, 32, 37, 39, 95, 96
Frictional coefficients, 27, 29, 36, 37
Frog, *see under Rana*
Frog skin, chloride fluxes in, 67
Frog skin, sodium fluxes in, 68

Griffithsia pulvinata, 64
  ion fluxes, 93
  membrane resistance, 73, 76
Goldman assumption, 5, 11
  flux equation, 6
  p.d. equation, 6

Halicystis ovalis, short-circuit current,
  68
Hodgkin–Katz equation, 6
Hydrodictyon africanum, 105

Ion activity, 60
  fluxes, 1, 6, 12, 74, 86
  selectivity, 56
  permeability, 6, 50
Ion exchange membrane, 34
  diffusion coefficients in, 35
  frictional coefficients of, 36, 37
  flux ratios in, 37, 39
Inhibitors of transport, 99, 101, 105
  table, 106

Length constant, 71
Local osmosis, 82
Loligo pealei, 51
  axoplasm, ion activity in, table, 60
  ion fluxes, 87
  membrane conductance and flux, 75
  membrane resistance, 73
  Na extrusion and O_2 consumption, 101

Membrane conductance, 11, 70
  and antibiotics, 41
  and flux, 12, 74
Membrane, fixed-charge, 8, 80
Membrane p.d., 6, 8
Membrane permeability, 50 ff
  Chara and *Nitella*, 54
  frog muscle fibres, 52
  marine algae, 56
  Sepia axons, 50
Membrane resistance, table, 73

Nernst equation, 4
Nernst potential, 63
Nitella, 52
  active transport in, 63
  Cl transport, 105
  electro-osmosis in, 82
  K flux and p.d., 96
  membrane resistance, 73
  Nernst potential in, 63
  p.d., 55
  vacuole concentrations, 55
Nitellopsis obtusa, 64
  tracer exchange, 91

Onsager's equations, 22

Partial conductance, 11, 74, 96
Partition coefficient, 5, 7
Photosynthesis and Cl transport, 105
  table, 106
Planck's assumption, 11, 78
Procambarus clarkii, 50
Punch-through, 78
  in *Chara*, 50

Rana pipiens, 88
Rana temporaria, single muscle fibres, 52
  ion activity in, table, 60

Rana temporaria, continued
  ion fluxes, 88
  membrane resistance, 73
  p.d., 53
Rectification by membranes, 77
Resistance coefficients (phenomenological), 22, 31
  in ion-exchange membrane, 36, 37

Sepia officinalis, giant axons from, 50
  ion fluxes, 87
  K flux and current, 75
  K flux and p.d., 95
  membrane resistance, 73
  Na and K fluxes, 101
  p.d., 51
Short-circuit technique, 68
Sodium transport, table, 100
Squid, *see Loligo pealei*
Streaming potential, 26
  in gall bladder, 84

Transport ATP-ase, 103

Ultrathin membranes, 40
  capacitance, resistance and water permeability, table, 42
Unidirectional fluxes, 9, 90

Valonia ventricosa, 69 ff
  fluxes, and ion distribution, 69
  membrane resistance, 73
  short-circuit current, 70
Valoniopsis, ion fluxes, 93